Contents

Acknowledgements

First of all I would like to thank everyone who participated in this research project – the social services departments, and in particular, all the older people who talked to me so openly and honestly.

I would also like to express my gratitude to Zetta Bear and Hazel Kemshall, who have given expert advice in regard to the research undertaken, but also emotional support when I have been affected by what I have heard during the course of project.

Melanie Whitehouse, administrative assistant, deserves special gratitude for her patience and tolerance in transcribing all the tapes.

Finally, very special thanks are due to Eric Sainsbury who has been invaluable in supporting me and commenting on the written drafts of this report.

Executive summary

Introduction

The abuse of older people is gradually gaining recognition in the United Kingdom, although in recent years the emphasis has been on the development and implementation of policy and procedures. This project set out to review the provision of services to victims of elder abuse and its findings have important implications for purchasers and providers in all sectors. The research, which was undertaken in three social services departments in the North of England, considers the life experiences of older women who have been victims of elder abuse, their past and present needs, and appropriate service provision.

Methodology

This study used a number of methods to identify the needs of older women. Monitoring systems were set up in the three departments in order to collate statistics on vulnerable adults, to identify older female victims for interview and to examine practices and outcomes. In-depth interviews were conducted with 27 female elder abuse victims and focus groups were run for over 300 older people. Social workers and other social care staff were interviewed and participated in focus groups. A number of older men were also identified as victims.

Statistics

- 186 cases were identified where a vulnerable adult had been a victim of adult abuse.
- 68% of these victims were older people.
- 52% of these victims were older women, aged between 60 and 99.
- 64% of female victims were aged over 75.
- 66% of known abusers were male, aged between 9 and 90.
- Physical abuse was the most common form of abuse identified by workers.

Themes

The main objective of the project was to gain an understanding of the different types of abuse and to identify the needs of victims. An insight was gained into victims' life-styles and the expectations of families and society in general, which often went some way to explaining why victims remained in abusive situations. Of those interviewed 14 victims had also been abused during earlier stages of their lives – seven were victims of child abuse; 13 of domestic violence.

In contrast to workers' reports which found physical abuse to be the most common, the most common forms identified by victims were financial and emotional abuse by family members. Victims described: the types of abuse, their definitions of abuse, its frequency, and their reasons for staying or leaving. Reference was also made to abuse by strangers; some victims had been abused by gangs and lived in fear because they perceived the police as indifferent.

Needs

Two chapters focus on 'needs' as defined by female victims and by workers. Victims' definitions are very specific, with emphasis on the need to talk, practical advice and information, appropriate housing and ongoing support. (In contrast workers focused very much on their own needs, apart from highlighting pious hopes for protection and safety.) It is clear that some current needs may have developed from past trauma and from the long-term effects of abuse. Skilful assessment is needed to identify the needs and the appropriate resources in order that the victim can heal and move on, both physically and emotionally.

Services

A broad range of services need to be readily available to help victims with their immediate practical and emotional needs. Longer-term help was erratic, and these services need further planning and coordination. Many services which are currently exclusively provided for younger victims could benefit older victims, but current practices do not encourage this flexibility in provision.

Conclusions

By the end of the project all three social services departments had policy statements in place; two had reviewed and rewritten their procedures during the course of the project. The policies provide workers with a sound working framework, but the quality of work is still sometimes poor and inconsistent. Because of other work pressures, elder abuse is often given very low priority; investigations may be rushed and long-term work with victims is unplanned and often cut short. It is not enough to simply produce a policy – there needs to be ongoing commitment to promoting good practice at field level and to address inadequacies in skills.

The inadequacies stem from a lack of knowledge and understanding about abuse and its long-term effects. There needs to be recognition that victims may need ongoing help and support for a long period of time. It can be helpful to make the distinction between short-term (assessment/investigation) and long-term work (protection/healing).

Agencies need to organise in-house training to cover:

- *Abuse*: definition/recognition/long-term effects
- *Assessment*: relevance of historical experience and current problems
- *Skills*: facilitating disclosure/listening/communicating
- *Methods*: use of techniques to work with older people in the long term

It was evident that many staff lacked skills in assessment; they were governed by the structure of their assessment forms rather than working in an holistic way to identify needs relating to both past and present events. Not enough time was spent discussing victims' earlier experiences and their bearing on current situations and problems. Workers felt pressurised by lack of time and consequently 'quick-fix' measures were often taken (for example, using residential care as a permanent solution without any follow-up to deal with ongoing problems). Insufficient time was given to planning and coordinating community resources for long-term work; cases were frequently closed when the presenting problem (ie, the abuse) had been alleviated, irrespective of ongoing needs.

There are many stages of healing – as there are for younger victims of abuse. Recognition that this can take years rather than months is crucial in planning resources for future intervention. Few victims had been offered the opportunity to work through their ongoing problems or their feelings about the abuse they had experienced. At a time when the role of social work is changing, other professionals and helpers may have a crucial role to play in long-term work.

There seems to be a stigma attached to older people which results in their low status within society as a whole but also within social care agencies. There needs to be recognition that work with older people can be stimulating and rewarding; that it is possible to effect change by setting goals and working with the victims at their own pace. Methods of working used for other service user groups can also be beneficial to older victims. Working with elder abuse can be stressful in the same way as child protection work, thus it is important that workers are committed to working with this service user group. Many workers were not motivated and morale was often very low. Agencies therefore need to ensure that they select staff who are committed to working with older people, and who can see that change can be achieved and is worthwhile regardless of age.

The services received by victims were variable, partly due to variations in workers' levels of expertise. Many unqualified staff lacked relevant knowledge or experience in assessment and in seeking out appropriate resources. There was an over-reliance on 'traditional' disposals (such as day centres, residential care etc). One of the most important findings of this project is that victims have a voice – that they know and can verbalise their needs. Thus, workers *must* communicate with and engage older people in their assessment to a greater extent, so that needs can be more accurately identified and appropriate services provided.

In conclusion there is a need for:

- Better selection of staff to work with victims
- Improvement in training
- More effective coordination at field level as well as in policy making
- Better definition of the skills required in short- and long-term work
- Better understanding of the relationships between short- and long-term work

1
Introduction

The abuse of older people is gradually being recognised as an important social issue in the United Kingdom and this will have important implications for all social care and health agencies (purchasers and providers) who work with older people. Research into elder abuse has been limited in this country and has focused on what constitutes elder abuse and definitions of abuse. There has been a concentration on prevalence, incidence and characteristics of cases (McCreadie, 1996). From early research undertaken in the 1980s and early 1990s, it was shown that the majority of elder abuse victims are female (Eastman, 1984; DoH, 1992). Small prevalence studies have been undertaken and there has been an emphasis on considering who is likely to be a victim or who is likely to be an abuser. However, little attention has been given to the needs of victims and the services they may require in both the short and long term.

There were indications in previous work (Pritchard 1989, 1990, 1995) that some older victims may have also experienced abuse earlier in their lives. The main aim of this project was to explore this further and to identify the needs of such victims. There has been very little research into how to work with victims of elder abuse in the long term. Research literature on survivors of child abuse (sexual abuse in particular) and domestic violence has been abundant, but the notion of older people as survivors has been largely ignored. Another omission has been the failure to recognise the links between child abuse, domestic violence and elder abuse, and the need for workers in these different specialisms to collaborate and learn from each other.

In recent years there has been renewed emphasis on *policy* – its development and implementation – within social and health care agencies; but the outcome has been to provide procedural frameworks for identifying abuse and for carrying out formal investigations. The present project set out to consider the *provision of services* to victims (from agencies in all sectors). In doing so, it moves the debate from policy and procedures to practices and professional competence. Service provision will be of growing importance as more older people are encouraged to remain in the community under the 1990 NHS Community Care Act.

The project's main aims were to:

1. Identify women who were victims of elder abuse
2. Carry out a small study to identify the extent to which victims of elder abuse have also experienced abuse earlier in their lives
3. Identify the types of abuse experienced (in childhood and adulthood)
4. Identify the needs of victims
5. Consider what resources and services should be provided to victims

---

Access

Gaining access to victims of abuse can be difficult as this is a very sensitive topic to research. Elder abuse is often well hidden and victims will frequently protect the abuser, especially if the abuser is a family member. Consequently, it can be difficult to access victims and even more difficult to encourage them to talk about the abuse they are experiencing. Thus, there has been very little qualitative research to date in this field due to the problems of getting victims to talk face-to-face.

In order to identify needs and appropriate services, the views of service users must be obtained and this was the fundamental aim of the project. It was important to obtain the views of older women rather than to make assumptions based solely on the views and assessments of professionals. The project planned to identify victims of elder abuse through records in social services departments: three departments in the North of England participated in the project between October 1997 and June 1999. These were based within metropolitan district/borough councils and for the purposes of this report will be referred to as Churchtown, Millfield and Tallyborough.

Churchtown and Millfield have had vulnerable adult/abuse policies in place since 1995 and 1994 respectively. While this research project was running, Tallyborough was working on a draft policy which became a working document in January 1999.

Ethics

From the outset it was important to give consideration to ethical issues. It was expected that confidentiality would be a major issue for the social services departments involved – this was particularly so in Tallyborough. Morale was very low in Tallyborough when the project began and social workers were suspicious of the motives of senior managers in participating in the project and suspected that there was a hidden agenda (that the researcher was evaluating practice for management's purposes rather than for the stated aims of the research project). There were also concerns about confidentiality and sharing information for the project in Churchtown and Millfield but not to the same degree.

The main issues in all three departments were related to completion of the monitoring forms devised for the project:

- Who owned the monitoring forms for obtaining information about victims and abusers (the research project or the department)?

- Who would have access to the data collected?

- Should victims and abusers be named on monitoring forms?

- Whether the monitoring forms should be used when there was only a suspicion of abuse (for example, when there was no definite evidence or where the worker, but not the victim, defined the situation as abusive).

- Whether the victim should be informed about the completion of monitoring forms.

In Churchtown and Tallyborough, the workers in the mental health teams were particularly resistant to completing the monitoring forms. However, all these issues were resolved by regular meetings between the researcher and senior managers, regular meetings with members of teams and the regular provision of information sheets about the research project, its aims and objectives and its progress. An agreed statement about confidentiality was produced.

One expectation was that workers would regard a research interview as an intrusion into the privacy of their own relationship with victims and hence may be unwilling to approach the victim. In fact, all the workers who were asked to approach their service users agreed to do this without hesitation and indeed were extremely helpful in organising the interviews. The issue of confidentiality and boundaries were discussed with the victim(s) at the beginning of each interview or at the start of meetings of the focus groups (see Chapter 2).

An important ethical issue was the risk of leaving victims without support after an interview had taken place. It was necessary to establish systems to check how the victim felt after the interview (the following day and a few days later) and providing immediate and appropriate support when it was needed. There were also concerns that where the victim was still living in an abusive situation (or the abuser had access to her), the victim could be at risk should the abuser find out that a disclosure has taken place.

Definition of abuse

Whichever aspect of abuse is being researched (in childhood or adulthood) a fundamental question arises: What is meant by the term 'abuse'? Definitions of abuse are often contested due to differing opinions about which behaviours are socially and personally acceptable and at what degree they become abusive. Much has been written in other studies about the difficulty in defining abuse and the problems this poses for researchers (McCreadie, 1996). The definition of elder abuse adopted for this project was taken from the national guidelines developed by the Social Services Inspectorate:

> Abuse may be described as physical, sexual, psychological or financial. It may be intentional or unintentional or the result of neglect. It causes harm to the older person, either temporarily or over a period of time. (DoH/SSI, 1993, p 3)

This definition was used in conjunction with the various policies and working documents available in the three contributing departments. A summary of definitions used in the departments is given in Appendix A.

The findings

This report summarises the main findings of the research project. After an overview of the methods used to obtain data, subsequent chapters will consider the themes which emerged from the interviews, the needs of older women both from the victims' and workers' perspectives, and finally the implications for service provisions, highlighting key areas of concern for purchasers and providers in all sectors.

2
Methodology

The main objective of this research project was to consider the prevalence of abuse of older women (both in community and institutional settings), some of whom may have also been victims of abuse earlier in their lives, and to find out how best to help them in regard to the abuse they have experienced or may still be experiencing. The methods adopted for the project needed to fulfil two main objectives:

1. To collect quantitative data regarding the victims, abusers, and types of abuse in the three social services departments.

2. To collect qualitative data about victims' experiences of abuse and to identify their needs, *both* for protection *and* in coming to terms with their abusive experiences.

As the project developed, multiple methods of data collection were used to explore the focus of enquiry. The purpose of this chapter is to explain why these methods were adopted and how they were used.

The research methods used

Historically, many researchers have used the positivist tradition in social science, that is, they seek causal explanations of violence by correlations of statistical data and favour hypothesis testing through *quantitative* methods. Feminist researchers lean towards interpretive and conflict theory, focusing on political, economic and cultural contexts. In pursuit of explanations and theory building many emphasise the importance and value of *qualitative* methods. Qualitative research is useful for certain types of exploration and is the method adopted for this study.

An important aspect of the research was to find out whether there were differences between needs as identified by victims and needs as identified by workers. Under the 1990 NHS Community Care Act workers have been encouraged to adopt a needs-led approach in their assessments. However, there may be differences in opinion about need between the various participants in specific situations. It was important therefore to find out whether victims were identifying the same need for resources as workers whose resources may be constrained by budgets and what is available locally. It was important to adopt methods which would collect data from both victims and workers in different settings.

Monitoring forms and questionnaires

In order to collect the qualitative data, it was necessary to identify a sample of victims for interview, thus, monitoring forms were used as the basic tool for collecting quantitative data, and to identify women suitable for interview. The monitoring forms were used to gain information about victims, abusers and the type(s) of abuse, and also provided material for a small quantitative exercise, the results of which are given in the following chapter.

The Vulnerable Adults Project had been set up in Churchtown in 1996. Monitoring forms had been designed for the Project after a survey of all the existing policies and guidance within local authorities in the UK relating to vulnerable adults, adult abuse and elder abuse (Pritchard, 1997). As these forms had been implemented successfully, it seemed appropriate to adopt them for this research project. The forms were modified slightly for each department participating in the project to incorporate local job titles and adapt to departmental computing systems. Four types of forms were sent out at the end of every month:

- managers' monthly monitoring form;
- fieldwork monitoring form;
- home care monitoring form;
- residential/day care monitoring form.

In Millfield and Tallyborough, where monitoring forms had not previously been developed or implemented, workers were first asked to complete questionnaires about all adult abuse cases they had worked on during the previous two years. These data were already available in Churchtown. Thereafter, they were asked to complete monitoring forms for every case they identified while the project was running.

Statistics from all three departments were collated on vulnerable adults and the definition from the Association of Directors of Social Services (ADSS, 1991) was used which defines a vulnerable adult as someone over 18 years of age falling into one of the following service user groups:

- elderly and very frail people;
- those who suffer from mental illness including dementia;
- those who have a sensory or physical disability;
- those who have a learning disability;
- those who suffer from severe physical illness (ADSS, 1991).

These definitions were circulated to all staff expected to be involved in completion of the monitoring forms: that is, staff within fieldwork teams, home care, residential and day care settings. In addition to cases involving abuse from known sources, information was also collected on abuse by strangers and on substantial self-neglect where this could have similar outcomes to abuse by others.

Identification of the group to be interviewed

It can be difficult to obtain a sample of abuse victims because of a number of issues:

- Confidentiality – agencies/workers may not be willing to disclose information about service users who are victims of abuse.
- Workers may not have raised the issue of abuse with the service user (even though recognising that abuse was occurring).
- The sensitivity of the topic – victims may not be willing to talk about their experiences because they are too painful or too threatening in their present circumstances.
- Victims may not be at an appropriate emotional stage to be able to talk about the abuse.
- Victims may still be living in abusive situations and fear repercussions if the abuser were to find out that they have disclosed information about the abuse which is taking place.
- Victims may be unable to communicate because of a particular disability or medical condition.

The group of older women who were to be identified for interview was not intended to be a representative sample of the populations in the three departments, but can be regarded as indicating the range of experiences and needs.

Several methods were used in identifying an adequate sample.

Monitoring forms

When a possible participant was identified, the worker was approached in the first instance. The criteria were that a victim should be a female, over 60 years of age, who had experienced elder abuse. If the worker thought it was appropriate to ask the victim to participate, the approach was made by the worker.

Identification by managers in day centres/resource centres

Once the project was running and information had been circulated, centre managers identified victims of elder abuse, who they thought might be willing to participate in the project. In these circumstances, the manager always asked the victim if she would like to be interviewed.

Focus groups/formal talks

Focus groups were run and formal talks given in day centres and resource centres (discussed in detail below) and some victims volunteered to talk further about their experiences away from the group setting.

Referrals from outside the social services departments

Workers within other organisations and projects approached the project about women who were not known to social services.

Approaches adopted

In the initial stages it was planned that the sample would be obtained solely from the monitoring forms. As the monitoring systems were being set up in Millfield and Tallyborough, it became clear that the number of women who could be approached for interview was very limited. The main reasons for this were:

- the worker did not want the victim approached;
- the woman had previously said to the worker that she did not want any action taken regarding the abusive situation or further intervention from social services;
- the worker had closed the case and felt it was inappropriate to return to the woman;
- the woman was confused or suffering from dementia and it was felt that an interview could be detrimental to her well-being;
- the woman had since died.

As the project developed, other methods were needed to obtain the sample. Managers of day centres and resource centres were approached directly, then the researcher attended team meetings to discuss the project with staff members. It was decided that with regular visits to the centres and by running focus groups or giving talks, further women would be identified for interview.

Focus groups/talks

Focus groups can serve a number of different purposes – either as a self-contained method in research studies or as a supplementary source of data (Morgan, 1997). For this project they were used as a method of identifying victims for in-depth interview, but also to gain data from a larger number of older women. The focus groups had small numbers of participants – usually between three and nine. In some situations, managers felt it was better to give a formal talk to a large group (50 to 60 people) and to invite discussion from the older people who attended. Informal talks were also given to small day care groups. In each situation the following subject areas were introduced for discussion:

- the meaning of the word 'abuse';
- types of abuse;
- violence and domestic violence;
- crime and punishment – past and present;
- harassment by gangs;
- availability and need for local services.

Over 300 older people who were attending day care facilities were met during the project.

In the final stages of the project, focus groups were run for workers in each department that had completed monitoring forms. They were asked to discuss 'the needs of elder abuse victims', so that comparisons could be made with the needs identified individually by women who had been interviewed, and collectively by those who had participated in the focus groups. A focus group was also organised for women who had been interviewed in order to validate the findings of the project.

In-depth interviews

The victims interviewed were identified in the following ways:

Monitoring forms	11
Day centre/resource centre	8
Focus groups	6
Outside organisation	2

To obtain data from victims themselves, in-depth unstructured interviews were conducted with 27 female victims of elder abuse. This method was thought to be the most appropriate; it allowed discussions to be initiated and guided by the researcher and topics and themes presented by the victim could also be developed by probing for additional detail. This type of interview allowed victims the opportunity to talk about their own perceptions of abuse and experiences, using their own terminology. The following broad subject areas were introduced, so that there was some consistency within and between the interviews:

• life history;
• definition of abuse;
• previous experience of abuse (in childhood/younger adulthood);
• experience of elder abuse;
• knowledge about other victims;
• what help/advice/support the woman received/needed at the time of abuse and currently;
• current needs.

A criticism of the validity of qualitative research has been that studies which use interviews as the main method of data collection rely on accounts from memory. It is recognised that people's feelings about events will change throughout a lifetime and situations may be perceived differently when years have passed by since the event happened. It was vital in this research to establish the victim's views on how they perceived what happened to them, but also to identify their needs, both in respect of past events and currently.

Most interviews were tape recorded with the permission of the respondent. A feature of qualitative research is that the focus of the inquiry may change as the research develops: it may be broadened or narrowed as appropriate. During the course of the project, some men asked if they could participate in the focus groups and this was agreed to by the women present. Managers also asked the researcher to talk to a number of men who were victims of elder abuse and subsequently in-depth interviews were conducted with six men. A summary of these findings will be published in a separate discussion document.

Telephone interviews

Telephone interviews were conducted with workers who had completed monitoring forms when:

- information was missing or unclear;
- the victim could not be interviewed;
- the case remained open during the running of the research project and the researcher needed to be updated.

During telephone interviews workers were asked about the current situation, and also about whether they knew of any history of abuse.

Other sources of qualitative data

Various documents can be used as another source of qualitative data. As part of the monitoring systems set up in each department, workers were asked to attach case conference minutes and protection plans to the monitoring forms. The researcher was also given access to files kept within the departments. Research diaries were also kept.

Analysis and validation of data

All the audio tapes from the interviews conducted were transcribed and then coded. The transcripts were read by an independent researcher to check the accuracy of coding and the analysis. A database was created to store data and computer software packages were used for the statistical analysis. As noted earlier, the findings of the project were validated by running a focus group for some of the interviewees. In addition, a summary of the findings was sent out to other interviewees for comment.

3

An overview of the quantitative findings: the extent of the problem

This chapter presents summary data collated from the monitoring forms used in the three social services departments who participated in the project. As discussed in the previous chapter, monitoring systems were set up in the departments in order to collate statistics about all vulnerable adults. The objectives were to collect information about the prevalence of abuse, to obtain details about victims and abusers and ultimately to identify older women who could be interviewed for the project.

Therefore, this chapter uses the workers' definition of abuse and not that of the service user. The following statistics have been compiled from monitoring forms which were completed during an 18-month period.

Table 1: Population of older people in the three localities		
	Total population	Population over 65
Churchtown	317,400	46,270
Millfield	218,550	30,160
Tallyborough	291,647	45,599

Victims

Vulnerable adults

In total, information was collected on 186 cases where a vulnerable adult was a victim of abuse. Table 2 and Figure 1 illustrate the breakdown between the departments.

Table 2: Vulnerable adults/adult abuse cases

	Number
Churchtown	64
Millfield	70
Tallyborough	52
Total	**186**

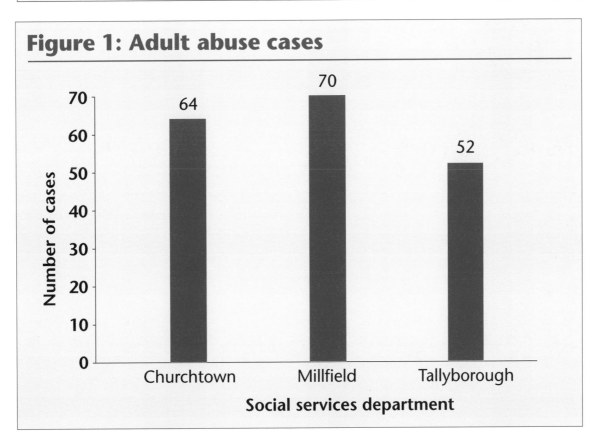

Figure 1: Adult abuse cases

Older people

definitions of the vulnerable adult men

It will be noted that older people constitute a high proportion of the total group of vulnerable adults. What is pertinent to this research project is the number of older people who were identified as abuse victims. The three departments had the following total number of referrals for adults over 65:

Table 3: Referrals of abuse victims aged 65 and over (1998/99)	
Number of referrals for adults over 65	
Churchtown	15,597*
Millfield	5,979
Tallyborough	16,832
Note: * Figure for Churchtown is 1997/98 which is the latest figure available.	

This study identified an older person as an adult over 60 years of age, rather than 65 years, in order to identify older women in receipt of a pension who may be victims of financial abuse. The numbers of older people identified constituted 68% of the total number of vulnerable adults. The monitoring forms identified older victims who were living in both domestic settings and residential care (19 in total).

The three departments are sufficiently similar to permit an aggregation of statistics from here onwards.

Table 4: Number of older people identified as vulnerable adults

	Total number	Number in residential care
Churchtown	50	13
Millfield	42	4
Tallyborough	34	2
Total	**126**	**19**

Figure 2: Victims of elder abuse (males and females)

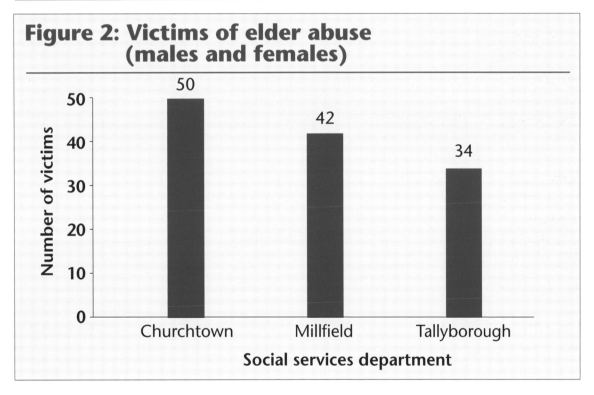

Gender

Of the 126 older people identified through the monitoring forms (see Table 2), 97 were women, that is, 52% of the total number of vulnerable adults. Earlier research in this country on victims of elder abuse has accepted that "the majority are female, over 80 and are dependent as a result of physical and mental incapacity" (Eastman, 1984, p 41). This project similarly found the majority of older abuse victims to be female (77%).

Table 5: Gender of abuse victims

	Female	Male
Churchtown	43	7
Millfield	30	12
Tallyborough	24	10
Total	**97**	**29**

Figure 3: Gender of elder abuse victims

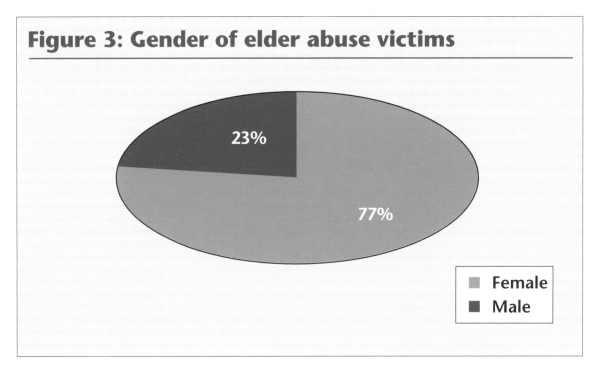

This is hardly a surprising finding: there are more females in the older population and women tend to live longer. However, when analysing why a woman is more likely to be a victim of abuse, other factors regarding gender should be considered such as oppression and socioeconomic factors (Aitken and Griffin, 1996; Dobash and Dobash, 1992).

Table 5 and Figures 3 and 4 show the divisions of older victims by gender between the three social services departments.

Table 6: Details of victims

Age	Number of abused older people	Number of abused older women
60-64	5	2
65-69	11	7
70-74	17	13
75-79	16	14
80-84	19	17
85-89	23	18
90-94	14	12
95-99	1	1
Not known	20	13
Total	**126**	**97**

Figure 4: Gender of victims (older people)

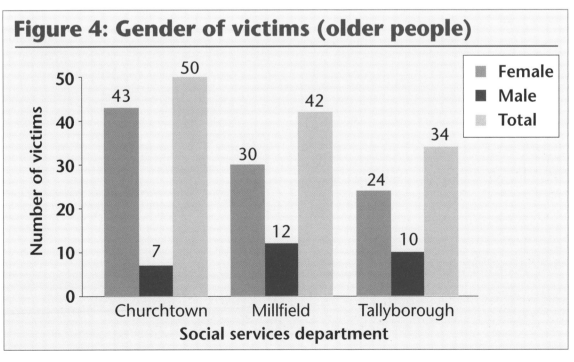

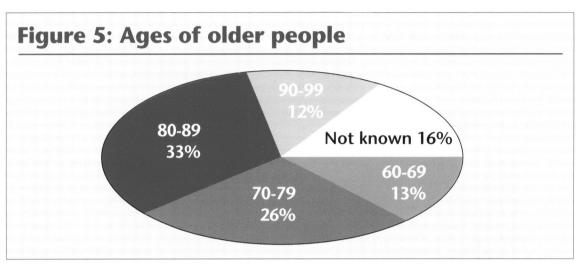

Figure 5: Ages of older people

90-99 12%

Not known 16%

80-89 33%

60-69 13%

70-79 26%

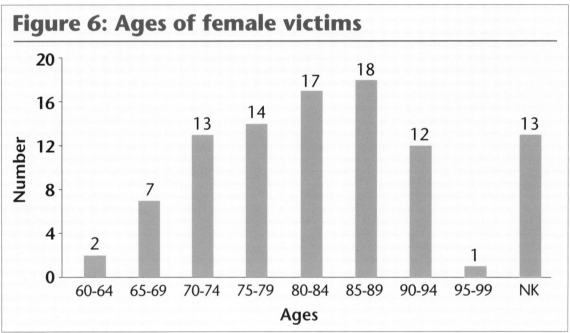

Figure 6: Ages of female victims

Ages

Age

The ages of victims ranged from 60 years to 99 years. The findings of this project also support the general assumption that the majority of victims are aged over 75 (see, for example, Eastman, 1984). The aggregate figures for the three departments are shown in Table 6 and Figures 5 and 6.

The 'older elderly' are considered to be those over 75 years of age. Among female victims in this project, 64% were aged over 75 years. This supports the expectation that although victims will be found in all age groups, there will be higher percentage in the older age groups.

Table 7: Physical, mental and medical problems

Condition	Number of victims
Dementia/memory loss	27
Stroke	12
Mobility problems	11
Mental health problems	8
Arthritis	7
Sight problems	7
Heart problems	6
Diabetes	5
Deafness/Hearing problems	4

Physical/medical conditions

In the past much emphasis has been placed on the physical or mental dependency of the victim as factors causing excessive stress for the carer, which may lead to physical or emotional abuse. Although this theory has been challenged, it was important to identify any specific health problems or disabilities that the victims may have. It became clear from the completed monitoring forms that elder abuse cases were often complex and few were direct outcomes of the carer's stress. Workers were asked to complete details of physical, mental or medical problems. The list of problems, both major and minor, was extensive because of the detail given by some workers. The main problems are identified in Table 7.

Other facts

The monitoring forms collected other information about the victims' backgrounds and circumstances. Out of the 97 women, 95 were white British, one was Dutch and one was Polish. No black elders were identified in any of the three departments. Twenty-five of the victims lived alone. Of the 72 victims who lived with someone else, 56 lived with the abuser(s).

Abusers

Getting information about abusers can be difficult for several reasons:

- the abuser may not be known;
- institutional abuse can involve groups of staff;
- the victim may not wish to disclose details;
- the worker has not asked for specific detail concerning the abuser.

Some workers were able to give detailed information about abuser(s), but others provided no details or only very scant information. What follows is a summary of information collected about 98 known abusers.

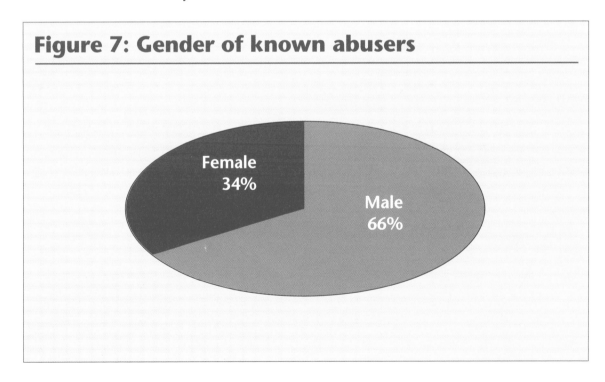

Figure 7: Gender of known abusers

Female 34%

Male 66%

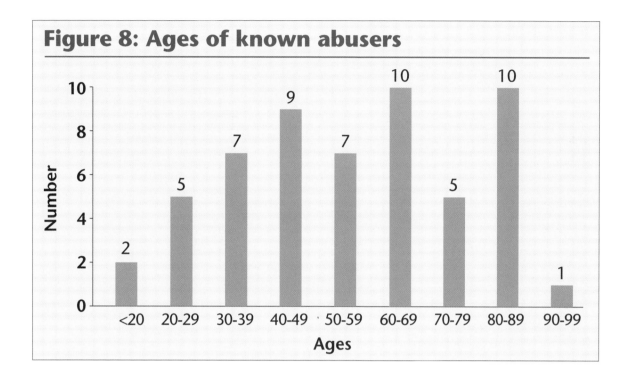

Gender

In early North American research into elder abuse, Gelles and Cornell stated:

> The abuser is typically identified as being female, middle aged and usually the offspring of the abused. (Gelles and Cornell, 1985, p 104)

This is based on an assumption that females do most of the caring for elderly people, when in fact, in this country, there is an equal divide between male and female carers. More recently research has shown that most abusers are male; this was borne out in this project where 66% of the abusers were male and 34% were female.

Age

The youngest known abuser was nine years old and the oldest was 90 years old. Of the known abusers, 45% were aged over 60 years and one third were in the two age groups 60-69 and 80-89.

Relationships

As discussed above, it was historically believed that females were more likely to care for dependent adults and that elder abuse may be the result of the carer's stress. This notion is far too simplistic. Many of the relationships between victims and abusers are extremely complex. Abuse identified through the monitoring forms took place in both domestic and institutional settings, therefore involving both personal and professional relationships. There were 12 cases where victims were abused by members of staff in institutional settings (for example, local authority day centre or older persons' home, private nursing home or hospital ward). In three cases an individual member of staff was identified, in the other cases allegations were made against groups of staff. In eight other cases, victims were abused by other service users in either a day centre or residential home.

Three cases of stranger abuse were identified and there was one case of self-neglect. The other cases which took place in domestic settings involved abusers who were known to the victims, either relatives, neighbours or friends. Table 8 summarises the relationships between victim and abuser and the 11 cases in which more than one abuser was involved.

Table 8a: Relationships between victims and abusers (multiple abusers)

Relationship of abusers	Number of cases
Relatives (male and female)	2
Son and daughter	2
Husband and son	2
Two sons and grandson	1
Niece and nephew	1
Brother and sister-in-law	1
Daughter and son-in-law	1
Neighbours (male and female)	1

Table 8b: Relationships between victims and abusers

Relationship of abuser	Number of cases
Son	21
Daughter	16
Husband	15
Residential staff (groups of)	8
Grandson	6
Relative (exact relationship not known)	6
Resident	6
Neighbours	3
Nephew	3
Brother	2
Friend	2
Partner (excluding husbands)	2
Bogus official	1
Daughter-in-law	1
Day centre manager	1
Day centre staff	1
Day centre service user	1
Granddaughter	1
Matron	1
Niece	1
Group of residents	1
Self	1
Sister	1
Sister-in-law	1
Son-in-law	1
Volunteer	1
Ward staff	1

Types of abuse

As has been found in previous research (Pritchard, 1995), victims frequently experience more than one type of abuse. Workers were asked to state which of the following categories the victims had experienced:

- physical
- emotional
- financial
- neglect
- sexual

Abuse was defined by worker not service user. Millfield and Churchtown had policies and guidance on vulnerable adults, which defined the categories of abuse (see Appendix A). Tallyborough was working on a draft policy and guidance, which became a working document during the course of the project. Some workers had previously been given training on adult abuse by the department and when the working document was launched all staff attended half-day briefing sessions.

Table and Figure 9 shows the number of victims who experienced different types of abuse. Physical abuse was the most common form: 58% of the older women experienced some form of physical violence. Substantial percentages experienced financial abuse (45%) and emotional abuse (43%). The figures for neglect and sexual abuse were much lower – 17% and 7% respectively. These two categories are relatively 'new' in that they were historically categorised as forms of physical abuse. Neglect can be emotional or physical, and can take a long period of time to identify. It is not surprising that few workers identified this category on the monitoring forms. Sexual abuse of older people is still very much a taboo subject and incredibly difficult to identify. Few older victims disclose sexual abuse for a range of reasons and workers often do not feel skilled enough to recognise the signs and symptoms. This research found that 47 victims experienced only one type of abuse; 36 of the victims experienced two types of abuse; 10 of the victims experienced three types of abuse; three of the victims experienced four types of abuse; one victim had experienced all five categories of abuse.

Table 9: Types and prevalence of abuse

Category of abuse	Number of victims
Physical	21
Emotional	2
Financial	14
Neglect	8
Sexual	2
Physical and Emotional	15
Emotional and Financial	10
Physical and Financial	5
Physical and Neglect	2
Emotional and Neglect	2
Financial and Neglect	1
Financial and Sexual	1
Physical, Emotional and Financial	7
Physical, Emotional and Sexual	1
Physical, Financial and Neglect	1
Emotional, Financial and Neglect	1
Physical, Emotional, Financial, Neglect	2
Physical, Emotional, Financial, Sexual	1
Physical, Emotional, Financial, Neglect, Sexual	1

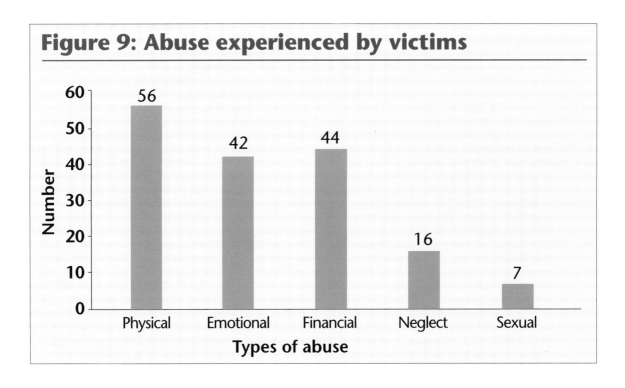

Figure 9: Abuse experienced by victims

4
Themes from the interviews: abuse in later life

During the project in-depth interviews were conducted with 27 women. Within the limited scope of this report, it is not possible to present the data on the continuity of abuse in earlier and later life (this will be the subject of a forthcoming discussion document). This chapter presents the common themes related to abuse in later life that arose during the interviews; specific needs and resources which were identified are

Table 10: Age of the women interviewed	
Age	Number of women
50+	1
60-64	5
65-69	0
70-74	1
75-79	5
80-84	7
85-89	2
90-94	4
95-99	2

presented later in Chapters 7 and 8. Appendix B contains information about the interviewees quoted in this and subsequent chapters.

The women

One of the criteria for interview was that the older woman should be aged 60 or over. One woman, Jessie, aged 54, was included in the project when the manager of a day centre asked me to interview her as she had recently been abused and had a very interesting history. The women were aged, therefore, between 54 and 98; the mean age being 79. The majority (75%) were aged over 75 years.

At the time of interview, two women were in nursing homes, six in sheltered accommodation and the remainder in their own homes. The interviews, which were conducted either at home or in day care settings, lasted between 30 minutes and four hours. Some victims were interviewed on more than one occasion. The women were asked to talk about:

- their life
- abuse – their definition
- abuse they had experienced
- their needs
- help and support

Abuse

The basic criterion for interview was that the older women had to be victims of elder abuse. Four of the victims had been abused by more than one person in later life, that is, they were 'multiple victims'. All interviewees were asked to explain what types of elder abuse they had experienced.

Financial abuse was cited as the most common form of abuse, with emotional abuse almost as prevalent. This contrasts with findings in previous work (Pritchard, 1989, 1990, 1995) and in the current project, that social workers, whether on monitoring forms or questionnaires, always indicate physical abuse as the most common type of abuse; their recording of emotional abuse has always been low. This may indicate that workers find it hard to identify emotional abuse or overlook it; either way they are at odds with the views and needs of the victims.

Table 11: Types of abuse

Category of abuse	Number of victims
Financial	20
Emotional	18
Physical	14
Neglect	3
Sexual	3

None of the women interviewed in this study became victims of abuse as a result of their carers being stressed (see discussion in Chapter 2). Those abused by carers were: Sarah, who was abused by her sister who was suffering with dementia (physical abuse and neglect); Beatrice, Bertha and Isabella were all financially abused by formal carers who were not related to them.

Financial abuse

Financial abuse was the most common form of abuse and took many forms. For example, money was:

- kept from women by their husbands;
- stolen by relatives/neighbours/formal carers/gangs/strangers;
- obtained by abusing the Power of Attorney.

A common complaint from workers is that it is difficult to work with abuse cases because often the victim does not see certain actions as abusive as it is the norm for them. What became very clear during the course of some interviews was that victims were very sure about what abuse meant to them, specifically in relation to how they had been financially abused by their husbands. They were absolutely sure they had been abused financially and this was a clear indicator that their attitudes had changed from when they were younger. Previously, they had accepted that 'you had to put up with it' or 'it was your lot in life'.

In later life they did not accept that their husbands had the right to hit them or deprive them of money. Once talking about financial abuse, the victims talked about the abuse in the past and the more recent incidents:

> "I couldn't rely on him for money or anything right from the start.... When I came out [of the maternity home] – they kept you in a fortnight in those days – he hadn't paid any bills. He'd bought a sports jacket out of the money so I had three weeks bills to pay when I thought I had only one. He'd arrange to buy something and I thought things must be looking up and then afterwards he said 'I'm short of so much you can pull something out of the bank. What have you got?'... Since he retired he never gave me a penny. My pension started at £120 a month and he took £80 off me towards the car." (Emma)

> "He always kept me short of money. I had to go out to work myself anyway, which I would rather do than be owing him." (Margaret)

> "I was always doing the paying out that all came out of my pension because he never gave me not one penny for 10 years. I never got any housekeeping or anything like that.... [I bought] food, but also bought curtains, carpets – not big carpets. I bought new carpet for the bathroom and bathmats, pots, pans, anything we needed renewing and utensils, bedding. I always bought all my own clothes right from the very beginning. I think he once bought me a coat and a dress when we were first married but I don't think he has ever bought me anything else since ... I used to pay half the telephone or especially all my calls if I have 'phoned [my son] in Australia, I paid for them. I didn't object to that because I thought well fair enough, but he used to charge me half rental." (Agnes)

Agnes also believed that her husband was financially abusing his daughter who had learning disabilities; he cashed all the benefits and kept them for himself. It was Agnes who bought her step-daughter all her necessities.

Some victims seemed more angry about financial abuse than physical abuse. One reason for this could be that the poverty and hardship they had had to endure were ongoing, and it also affected their children. Depriving a woman of money was a method of keeping control and limiting what she could do, which explains further why women felt unable to leave abusive situations.

Where financial abuse occurred only in later years, the victim had usually experienced theft of money and possessions either by people they knew or by strangers. The amounts involved varied considerably. Georgina had been conned by a man who called at her house and took £110; in other cases (Isabella and Gertrude) a relative or neighbour had taken Power of Attorney for amounts totalling over £50,000. Isabella's nephew had cashed her insurance policies and also regularly took money from her; with the proceeds he bought a house in Bridlington. Beatrice and Bertha, who were abused by formal carers, did not know exactly how much money had been stolen because the money had been taken in small amounts over a long period of time; sometimes the cash was taken from in the home, while shopping or from a bank account to which the abuser had access.

It is recognised that the recurring abuse often occurs because the abuser has a particular problem. Four victims were abused physically and financially by their grandsons; three of whom had brought the boys up from infancy. Florence, Joan and Irene's grandsons needed money to finance their drug use. Irene was aware that her grandson, who came to live with her after being in prison, and his friends were using drugs:

> "It's them drugs. They do it for a laugh. There is gang of them doing it. I know what they are like. I have money taken…. They rob old people for drink and drugs." (Irene)

Florence and Joan were not aware initially of their grandsons' drug addictions. They were both having problems with their grandsons and being physically abused but would not disclose this to their respective social workers. It was only while Joan was in hospital after attempting suicide and Florence was in temporary care that the police and family members found used syringes in the attics of the women's houses:

> "I couldn't believe what they found in the house. I couldn't believe
> it.... They found needles all over ... there were some that were used
> ... what they threw out was disgusting." (Joan)

Joan and Irene talked at length about what they had lost; the boys had
stolen huge amounts of money and possessions to sell on:

> "He must have told me a pack of lies. He was after money all the
> time for this and that.... He has stolen the television, pension, two
> new cardigans that I have never had on, clothes, a nice anorak and a
> car coat, suits he will have sold. He took all my jewellery, a gold
> chain that [husband] bought me for my 21st, two plain gold chains.
> He took a chain that I had bought for my 40th wedding anniversary
> with orange stones. He took my engagement ring. He took a ring
> which was left by my grandma that was 22-carat gold and had a
> ruby in." (Joan)

> "He took my camera, purse and keys. The week my husband died
> he took £80 and £20 from my purse." (Irene)

Florence, Irene and Joan had previously denied that their grandsons had
physically abused them, even though there was evidence of this. Irene
was interviewed six weeks after she had been badly battered by her
grandson and two sons; she was still covered in bruises on her face and
arms. The police had been called out but she refused to press charges.
Joan was adamant that her grandson had never hit her, but openly
talked about the fact that he regularly grabbed her around the throat:

> "It frightened me to death because he used to go and get hold of me
> like that [puts hands around her throat]. I said 'Give over you are
> going to choke me', and he used to shout and ball.... He hasn't ever
> hit me.... It used to hurt. I used to say 'One of these days you'll
> strangle me'.... If he had hit me I would have called the police but
> you see he never hit me.... I was terrified of him." (Joan)

As noted earlier, some victims do not see certain actions as physical
abuse. Joan would not accept that attempted strangulation was a
physical assault, probably because she still found it difficult to accept

what her grandson had done to her; victims spoke about feeling 'ashamed' when admitting what a relative had done to them.

Daphne was abused financially by her granddaughter who was a drug user. Over a period of time Daphne noticed that different amounts were missing from her pension, a special envelope in which she was saving for a holiday and from her purse:

> "I started noticing that my money was going down quickly.... I started to put the money in the bank so she couldn't touch it ... when she got my cheque book there were 14 blank stubs ... she had cashed and falsified my signature ... she was hitting cannabis and that is where all the money was going." (Daphne)

After a visit from the bank manager, the bank gave Daphne her money back (£931) because the manager said: "It was their fault for not checking the signatures ... they were obvious forgeries."

In other cases, victims felt a sense of duty towards their offspring and felt that they had to help them. Martha described her son as:

> "... a bit of an alcoholic ... he had been to the pub ... there were a lot of lads been breaking in. I had been sat watching the television and they got into the kitchen, seen my purse and went in my back and took money out.... They are a gang of thieves. It's as though you have been raped in a way. Coming into your house. Terrible. An awful feeling. He has been coming in drunk at night." (Martha)

Martha rationalised what her son did to her by talking about his problems which were that he was an alcoholic, did not work because he 'has disabilities' and his son, aged 21, had recently died:

> "... he went to call him up the next morning and he was laid dead in his bed with his arm out. It has been a shock for him.... He's supposed to have hayfever. He has had some of those tablets in the house and he took 60 of them."

Martha was also another multiple victim because she was being financially abused by her daughter who managed her bank account:

> "What I don't like about her, she thinks what I get it's hers. She takes it to the bank what I save now and I have never been able to have anything myself now. I used to go and shop and get something. I can't.... They have got a new car ... and I can't go nowhere and they are going on holiday all the time. They go abroad all the time and I am stuck here like this.... She knows where my savings are but she doesn't like me getting any. She doesn't want me to get a lamp. I'm going to do. It's my money. I'm going to get one. She's got everything."

Other women felt a maternal duty to provide for sons who were unemployed and so justified the abuse. Ethel had bought her son a car because he was unemployed and she believed it would help him "to get about to do some jobs". Eva, who was regularly threatened by her son, rationalised it by saying:

> "I know that if I don't give him money when he asks for it there will be a row.... There has been the recession and jobs have been pretty scarce so I have given him small amounts for things and clothing." (Eva)

Emotional abuse

Workers appear to find emotional abuse difficult to define, but victims found it very easy to talk about the 'mental cruelty' inflicted on them. Victims of domestic violence tended to talk about the way their husbands had abused them in the past and more recently:

> "Everyday he was suggesting I wasn't right in my head that I had forgotten to do something and I knew I hadn't." (Emma)

> "I love gardens and flowers, but with my husband he doesn't like gardening. But yesterday I really felt it when he said how lovely my bowl of crocuses were because I planted them the year before last and they might have multiplied. They were all colours – yellow, white, purple and striped – and he said how nice they are now. And yet before he was always getting on to me about them.... That's the way I look at it. A bit of mental cruelty." (Agnes)

The emotional abuse was often very subtle and was a way of controlling the victim. The abuser often made the victim feel she was 'useless' or 'inadequate' so that her self-esteem was very low, for example, Agnes' husband constantly told her that she had "no brains".

When talking about this type of abuse most of the victims talked about their fear and how they felt threatened. Often it was as though they were reliving that fear; they visibly shook and looked terrified as they were recounting what had happened, some broke down at this point.

Neglect

Neglect can be either emotional or physical. Isolation is also a form of neglect. For workers this is difficult to identify, because it is often subtle and the abusers may not allow the worker to see the victim alone. Isabella was particularly vulnerable because she had been in a mental institution for 20 years and found it difficult to stand up for herself. She was physically abused by her husband, who she described as "a bad one", but then went to live with carers who kept her isolated in the conservatory:

> "It was awful she wouldn't let me do anything ... never went out ... they used to shout a lot." (Isabella)

Vera was kept virtually a prisoner by her husband when she became ill and for seven-and-a-half months she was physically neglected.

> "He wouldn't get a doctor ... I had to crawl on my hands and knees up the stairs to get into bed." (Vera)

She believes that he was trying to kill her and on admission to hospital it was thought she would die. She was suffering from malnutrition and dehydration. Vera described what her life had been like during those months when she was kept isolated:

> "He knew what he was doing ... you could see the smile on his face ... the worst thing was when he left me in a cold bathroom ... I was trapped in the bath for four hours ... he threw me in two pillows and a sheet ... it was just the expression he used to get on his face. It used to tell you what he was aiming to do.... [My son] came in at 11 and it was thanks to him that he got me out of the bath."

Ethel was regularly 'abandoned' at the day centre by her son. She resented being 'dumped' as she put it, because she wanted to be at home. Her son would bring her to the centre later than everybody else and instead of picking her up at around 3.30pm, he often left her there until 10.00pm. Ethel used to get very angry and agitated about this and on occasions when her son arrived to collect her she would wet or soil herself.

Sarah is severely disabled and needs help with all personal care. She was neglected by her sister who was her main carer but suffered with Alzheimer's disease. Sarah argued that it was not her sister's fault that she did not look after her properly; her sister was not capable of providing the care she needed and on occasions became violent towards Sarah.

Not being involved in major decision making was considered to be neglect by others. For example, Stella was feeling very anxious about moving to a bungalow which had been seen by her husband and the rest of her family, but not herself. Agnes felt that she had been pushed into making a hasty decision about moving into a nursing home by her son and social worker.

Sexual abuse

Sexual abuse of older people is a taboo subject and it can be extremely difficult for the older women themselves to talk about sexual matters. However, three victims (Harriet, Jessie and Vera) were able to talk about the sexual abuse they had experienced. Staff suspected that Ethel was being sexually abused by her son, however there was no firm evidence and Ethel certainly did not disclose this in her interview.

Harriet was adamant that she had been raped by a man living in the same sheltered accommodation complex. Harriet was slightly confused and hence very few people believed her, including her social worker, the police and her family (although later her son became convinced that she was telling the truth). Staff in the resource centre said that they did believe that Harriet had been sexually assaulted in some way. She gave exact details about what had been done to her and her story was consistent over a long period of time:

"I had never spoken to the fellow. I had seen him about but I had never spoken to him and it came as a shock when he followed me into the flat and did what he did.... He started to undress me and I thought well it's a funny thing to do to come in and start to do anything like that. I said, 'you don't do that here', and so ... [pause] I really forgot what was said really but he never took any notice of me to stop doing what he did. It went right to the finish [pause] I was all upset inside. I was really upset." (Harriet)

The social worker said that she did not believe Harriet was capable of having sex standing up (which is what she alleged) and felt a lot of sympathy towards the alleged abuser, as did the police. The social worker also thought it was 'odd' that Harriet did not get upset when talking about what had happened and that she had not called for help immediately. Harriet said:

"I was really frightened that he would do something. I was frightened that he might hit me, or something like that, if I told anybody."

She kept calm because this was how she had always coped; it was a strategy that she had developed. The current attack may have triggered memories of how she had been threatened in the past. Harriet returned to live in the same complex and months later another woman claimed to have been raped but again nothing was proven. The alleged abuser then moved out of the complex.

Vera was forced to have sex by her husband and earlier in life she had considered this to be his right; later she realised it was abuse. Jessie talked about the telephone calls she has received from her brother which she defined as sexual abuse:

"He used to abuse me on the 'phone sexually, saying 'How many times have you had it?', and, 'You're gay because you haven't got a fellow'." (Jessie)

Reasons for abuse

The victims spent much of their interview time giving details about how they had been abused both recently and in earlier life, but other important themes emerged. Victims tried to provide explanations for their abuser's behaviour. Alcohol was mentioned in relation to violence and causing financial problems.

> "He used to drink a lot. He used to go out Friday nights and come home drink and he used to be up all night. Sometimes I had to run out of the house." (Margaret)

> "And his family used to drink so there is no wonder [son] is like that. He [husband] used to take bottles to work with him to drink, so that is where the drinking has come from.... He did use to go mad a bit at times with drink. He used to come in and throw things at the walls. That was drink." (Martha)

Vera had been kept short of money because her husband "used to be a big time gambler on the horses".

Deciding to leave

Victims who had left an abusive situation were asked what had ultimately made them take the decision to leave. Illness had caused some of them to reach a very low point and to feel unable to take anymore:

> "I was so poorly, physically and mentally exhausted. I just knew I couldn't go on anymore.... I thought until he bashes me and I go into hospital, or else he kills me, and then they'll do something, and I thought well I can't wait that long." (Emma)

> "Well I was feeling very low, very depressed. It had got to me to such an extent over the last few years I had gradually got lower and lower. I felt I didn't want to live anymore. I wasn't even living. I was just existing and he didn't do anything to help. He still carried on going out dancing and enjoying life, but not giving any consideration to me." (Agnes)

Vera believed that her husband had tried to kill her by starving her and thought he would try again if she returned home:

"It was a mixture of fear of doing it again only this time succeeding ... doing it in a more rash way ... and the other was hate.... I hate him for what he has done to me and what he has done with my life. I had no life with him." (Vera)

Some women felt that the only way to leave the situation was by attempting suicide. Hilda and Lilian had overdosed on numerous occasions and Joan had attempted suicide once.

"I thought, Sunday night I have nothing to live for. I was going to go out and jump in the river and then I thought 'No, I'll stop where I am comfortable and take tablets', and I did. I took everything I could lay my hands on and I was hoping that I would go ... [the doctor] told me that they had only just got me in time. But I said 'Why? I didn't want to live, I wanted to die', and he said, 'Would you do it again?', and I said, 'Yes I would if I had got the chance'. I said 'I haven't nothing to live for'." (Joan)

Agnes had also contemplated suicide:

"I got lower and lower, but still I was trying to keep the peace all the time. I think it was eating into me, the unhappiness. I was really unhappy. I felt I just wanted to die." (Agnes)

Loss and bereavement

Victims also wanted to talk about the many types of loss they had experienced in their lives, including:

- childhood
- living life as they would like
- contact with children
- bereavement
- limbs

Women who had been abused early in their lives felt that they had had to grow up too quickly and had never experienced a 'proper' childhood. Likewise those who had been abused by their husbands for years felt that they had wasted their lives. All the women interviewed had experienced bereavements: siblings (early and late life), parents, miscarriages, their own children, grandchildren and husbands.

Vera's husband had promised her that he would always keep her pregnant; Vera explains this as his way of controlling her. She had 10 pregnancies, but only two sons survived. During the interview Vera talked at length about the miscarriages and the babies who had died. She is still distressed that her husband had buried one son "in a pauper's grave", and because he threw away the papers she has no way of knowing where the baby is buried. When Vera suffered her first miscarriage she was living in an area of Scotland which was new to her:

> "I lost the baby at 12 weeks.... He [husband] didn't even come to the hospital to see if I was alright ... I was just left there and after three days I was discharged and I knew nothing about the bus services or anything and I had to find my way back up town and as I walked in his mother shouted to him, 'She's back', and it was as though I was nothing." (Vera)

Other losses followed:

> "I used to make sure my boys were well fed and I was literally living on a diet of cornflakes and milk which ended up causing malnutrition ... I went into labour on 9th October 1966 and I lost the baby. It was a girl. She was only 1lb 2oz. I have lost eight. I had a girl in January 1965. As you know I have two sons living but there was a miscarriage between those two. In 1960 I miscarried in the August because he made one promise to me and that was that he would kick me into the fireside and I would always be pregnant. So he made the threat and carried it out but what he didn't realise my life was on the line all the time ... I had four pregnancies from January 1965 until October 1966."

Agnes, Beatrice, Dorothy, Gertrude, Isabella, Lilian and Martha had all experienced the death of a child. Other victims had lost their children in other ways. Hilda's children had been taken from her when they were very small; her daughter has never known her mother. Hilda has seen her daughter at relatives' funerals but has not spoken to her. Jessie had a daughter adopted, but recently traced her and is now in regular contact with her. Joan and Jessie have little contact with their sons.

> "[After attempted suicide] they rung him from the hospital and told him how poorly I was and do you know what he said? He said, 'I have got married again and I have a life of my own', and he never even asked how I was or came to see me." (Joan)

> "I saw him last year. Sometimes there is no contact in three or four months. His favourite saying is 'I have forgotten', and he even forgot my address for a Christmas card and it hurts but you have to get on with it." (Jessie)

Another common loss was contact with family members. This was either because the relatives lived in another part of the country or the victim was housebound. Sarah was particularly upset by this as she had had a large number of step-brothers and step-sisters and even though relatives lived nearby they did not visit or take her out.

Crime in the community

It was not only victims who had been abused by strangers and gangs who talked about crime in the community. Many respondents felt this to be a very important issue when asked to talk about what abuse meant to them. They knew neighbours who been burgled or mugged and were conscious of the fear of crime:

> "You didn't have all this going on. No one breaking in because we could go to bed and leave the door unlocked, but look at it now it is going on all over. There is women stood at the bus-stop with purses in their hand. They just ride up and grab the purse. There is a woman who lives over there. She had been to church with her mates. Grabbed her bag from her, knocked her flying." (Martha)

Eva had decided to remain living with her abusive son partly because of her fear of being alone:

> "I should hate to be in the house on my own because of being afraid on my own. Someone breaking in and it happens all the time." (Eva)

Jessie had been mugged in the street and the fear of being attacked has remained with her:

> "I was a gibbering wreck, I couldn't do a thing. I couldn't even pick the 'phone up. It has left me terribly scared because I am still looking behind me all the time.... It took me two hours to go out the first time ... I won't even go down there on my own in this [wheelchair] I get a taxi now.... When I am outside I feel very vulnerable." (Jessie)

Regrets

All the victims who had left an abusive situation were glad they had done so, but still had some regrets. Agnes spoke for all when she said:

> "I think I have wasted all those years. I wish I hadn't have married him in the first place."

5
Needs from the victims' perspectives

This chapter describes the needs of the victims as identified by older women themselves. This information was obtained during the in-depth interviews with victims and during the focus groups run for older women. During the in-depth interviews women were asked about their current and past needs. Victims, who had experienced abuse earlier in their lives, spoke of the fact that no help had been available, so they were asked to consider with hindsight what would have helped them at that point in their lives and whether the needs were different when they wanted to leave an abusive situation later in their lives. This chapter looks at:

- past needs
- needs when leaving an abusive situation
- needs having left an abusive situation
- current needs

Past needs
Nowadays people are encouraged to talk about how they feel and to ask for help when it is needed. Years ago the situation was very different. It was expected that if you had a problem you kept it to yourself. It is extremely difficult for people to leave abusive situations; much has been written about the difficulties faced by women living in domestic violence situations. To date little has been written about what it was like for abused women years ago when attitudes were less open.

Women often felt that there was no escape and that they had to put up with whatever life gave them. Victims often indicated that they could not discuss problems with family or friends:

> "Our silly mothers – my mother said it to me, 'You make your bed you must lay on it'." (Emma)

> "... my mother was on her own. All my other family were married off and happy on their own. I didn't want to bother nobody else. I just stuck it out ... I didn't tell anyone for ages." (Margaret)

Loyalty is a major factor in explaining why women chose to stay in abusive situations; even later in life it continued to have a powerful impact and women felt that they had to protect the abuser because he or she was a family member. Margaret felt guilty talking about the abuse she had experienced. After each vivid account of violence, she asked the same question: "It is alright to talk about him now he's dead, isn't it?" She felt that her husband was still controlling her from the grave; when she told him she would leave he repeatedly threatened her:

> "He said, 'You'll never be happy because I'll haunt you, I'll follow you around'." (Margaret)

Victims need to be able to talk about their abusive experiences without feeling disloyal or guilty: to disclose what actually happened and to talk about their feelings from the past and how they are feeling now. Some victims referred to the fact that "it is different nowadays", but even though they acknowledge that younger people talk more openly, it is still hard for them to do so.

All interviewees or participants in the focus groups were asked if they had ever known anyone else who had lived in a domestic violence situation; very few had because 'people didn't talk about it'. Consequently, women who were abused felt isolated and felt that no one would believe them if they spoke about it.

For some victims it had been important to maintain the reputation of the abuser or the family.

> "I didn't tell anyone for ages. I put up with it because I didn't want people to know that he was like he was." (Margaret)

The shame of disclosure is as significant now as it was in the past. The police were called out to Irene on several occasions when she was badly beaten by her two sons and grandson, but she refused to press charges.

Irene lives in a close-knit community and was ashamed that the police had been seen coming to the house:

> "We have never had the police – me and my husband. We have never done anything." (Irene)

Needs when leaving the abusive situation

Women frequently stayed in abusive situations in earlier life because they had nowhere to go and no means to support themselves and their children. Their needs then were not dissimilar from the needs they have more recently experienced as victims of elder abuse. Several victims stated that they had thought about leaving an abusive situation for a long time, but were held back by lack of knowledge about where to go for help. One of the major needs cited in this research was for practical advice and information, but, initially, someone to talk to about their situation.

The need for people and to talk

Victims can feel very isolated when living in an abusive situation, especially if the abuser will not permit contact with the outside world. This was the situation for many of the victims interviewed. What they needed most was for someone to tell them how they could leave the situation safely.

Of paramount importance was the need for someone to:

- listen
- believe what is disclosed
- give practical advice
- organise the 'escape' and obtain possessions
- be trustworthy
- maintain privacy

Victims were questioned about who would be an appropriate person. They appear to have found people to do this in different settings. For example, Emma had disclosed to an acupuncturist at the GP's surgery:

> "[The acupuncturist] said, 'Well, I'll have to write a report to your doctor', and I knew she had. She did that and my doctor evidently had reported to the social services and she had also alerted the police.... So down they came – four police cars with policemen and policewomen and the social worker teamed up with them and they came in ... I came out just as I am now in my slippers and the lot. They went back and got my handbag for me." (Emma)

In other situations, the victim has been able to leave home for another reason, perhaps an admission to hospital, and then decided not to go back. Vera had suffered extreme physical violence from husband all through her 42 years of marriage:

> "... never knew what to expect and if a day went by and I didn't get a punch or a head butt then it was something unusual." (Vera)

When she became ill with a urine infection and breathing problems, he did not seek medical help. She was neglected over a period of six months. She was kept in the lounge and only had a spoonful of mashed potato to eat each day. On admission to hospital it was thought she would not live through the night:

> "My nightdress had to be cut off me because the sores were bleeding. I had them under the breasts ... in the groin ... I needed six units of blood and they were putting drips of antibiotics into me and giving me B12 injections because every part of my body was at the lowest it could be."

If victims have been threatened by the abuser they are often petrified of verbally disclosing the problem and find other ways of communicating. Lilian was abused physically and financially by her son, who lived nearby. One morning when the home care assistants came in she gave them a note which said: 'My son hurts me. Get me out'. This was reported immediately; a social worker came and Lilian was taken from the house and found an emergency placement. Lilian continued to write notes about the abuse but still refused to talk about it. She would talk normally about anything else, but returned to the notepad every time the subject returned to the abuse from her son. Lilian was terrified of her son and the possibility that she had disclosed about what he had been doing to her. Lilian felt she was not betraying her son when writing about the abuse; it is seen as a way of 'not really telling'. Emma had also used notes to tell a social worker who visited her husband what was happening because he would not let her talk to anyone:

> "I used to write notes to her to tell her exactly what was going off. She got in touch with this other social worker and eventually [new social worker] wrote me this note. Said would I meet her at the surgery at 3 o'clock on this Thursday afternoon ... I knew I wouldn't make it for 3 o' clock, if I could have got out at all." (Emma)

Workers need to be aware of the victim's fears and consider using a variety of methods to facilitate disclosure. Some victims keep diaries, as Vera did, and may be willing to share them with a social worker.

Joan was abused by her grandson who was using and selling drugs; she became unable to cope and attempted suicide. Ironically, her grandson came in during the evening, which he did not usually do, and got her to hospital. While in hospital, Joan eventually felt able to talk to a psychiatrist about what she had been going through and made the decision not to return home:

> "It was a long time before they got anything out of me. I felt I couldn't ... I sort of opened out to someone I didn't know rather than those I had been used to." (Joan)

It should be noted that, as in many ambivalent situations, some victims are more ready to tell a stranger rather than someone they know. Thus workers need to be aware of signals that a victim needs or is ready to talk; this may happen at a time of crisis or when the victim is feeling that they have had enough. In Joan's case the psychiatrist asked some very direct questions and acknowledged how difficult it must have been to be abused by a family member. Joan had not been able to open up to her social worker or family in the same way.

Practical advice and information

Despite current emphasis on non-discriminatory practice, it seems that ageist attitudes and the belief that it is 'too late' sometimes prevent older women being offered useful advice. This study found that older and younger women have similar practical needs in leaving abusive situations. The women interviewed had chosen to leave their situation and were clear about the sort of advice they needed. However, they were far from clear about their rights and entitlements. This appeared to be associated with traditions of self-reliance in hardship and of independence from benefits.

Ironically, their apparent past independence and self-reliance (or independence of the family as a group) had, in a sense, made them easier for their abusers to control. It was important to offer advice and information in ways which gave them a sense of taking control of their own lives. Money was particularly important. Victims had many questions regarding financial affairs, such as how to access money held in a joint bank account and how much rented accommodation would cost. Knowledge was limited about the benefits system. A major worry about leaving an abusive situation was whether they would be able to survive financially, for example, who would pay the rent.

A common criticism from the victims was the length of time it took to get things sorted out, especially benefits. The application forms were 'too complicated' and most victims needed help with completing them. Emma was 80 years old and suffering with arthritis and emphysema when she left her husband. She had an emergency placement in a resource centre before being offered sheltered accommodation. She was worried about her financial situation and forced herself to go out to get information. She had just moved into a flat when the interview took place:

> "I can't get about. Yesterday I thought I would try it. I took it steadily and I managed but every seat I came to I had to have a sit until I got into town.... This flat is costing me more than I get. I only get £37 a week and the flat is £54. When I went up town the other day to the Citizens' Advice Bureau they sent me down to the DSS. She gave me forms to fill in which I filled in to the best of my ability and I took them across yesterday.... Then I went to pay my rent and then the bank is right alongside the Post Office and they didn't have my cheque book with my new address in. There is a cheque book at home. The only way I'm going to go back is with a policeman." (Emma)

Vera had to wait three months for the DSS officer to visit her at home. Her claim was complicated by the fact that her son, who has learning disabilities, worked and was expected to pay rent. Vera had to go to court about getting money from her husband. When the officers *did* visit they were helpful and told Vera she was entitled to other benefits; but the initial delay at a time of personal crisis was damaging.

Solicitors are sometimes needed for advice on a range of matters, for example, applying for court orders (such as those under the 1996 Family Law Act and 1997 Harassment Act), the division of money and assets, and the pros and cons of divorce – how easy it would be to obtain, how long it would take, how money and assets would be split. Making a will was also important to ensure that the abuser would not inherit anything if something should happen unexpectedly. Victims felt a sense of urgency to sort this out:

> "I had to go into hospital for a week and I wanted to see the solicitor before I went in there to make a will. Not that I had much to leave, but I certainly didn't want him to get what I had got." (Emma)

The cost of legal fees was also an unknown and presented yet another worry. It became clear that all this information should be made readily available and this is discussed further in Chapter 7.

An important finding at this stage is that these are issues that tend not be explored by social workers and other helpers, despite their emotional importance. In the focus group which considered the project's findings, women commented that they had eventually got the advice they needed but that it happened too slowly. They also felt that they had too many people from different agencies visiting them and that they therefore had to repeat their story too many times. They felt that it would have been more helpful to have only one person visiting them, who "would be like a link person" and who could work on their behalf with the other relevant people and agencies.

Place of safety
A fundamental need for all victims is for a place of safety. If a victim suddenly decides to leave an abusive situation, agencies need to be able to provide emergency placements immediately. Victims should not be

told that they have to wait (maybe days or over a week) while somewhere is found. In Churchtown, resource centres have been crucial in providing effective emergency placements and in subsequently working very closely with the victim (in conjunction with the social worker) to find long-term accommodation. Emma planned her escape and was escorted out of her home by the police and social worker. She and her son, Stephen (aged 50 with learning disabilities) went to stay temporarily in a resource centre. Emma talked in interview about how the abuse had affected her son and about the positive effects the stay in the resource centre had on them both:

> "We were there eight weeks. They are marvellous there. They are all so kind. They couldn't do enough for us. It's like a first class hotel. The meals were marvellous and Stephen came out of his shell. My sister couldn't believe the change in him. But we had been so subdued, and Stephen, when he got up in the morning, he used to walk around the bungalow and I had to call him in for his breakfast. He knew what was going on because he would shout 'Stop it. Shut up'. He would sit and wait for me on the telephone seat in the hall, for me to get up and get hold of me." (Emma)

Emma went to live in sheltered accommodation and Stephen was placed permanently with carers. Victims sometimes have responsibility for adult children which is another reason why they may decide to stay in the abusive situation. Consequently, another important issue can be finding suitable accommodation for the dependent adult.

Vera also had a son with learning disabilities. After admission to hospital following gross neglect, she said she would not go back. She was given a council house in a new area where her son came to live with her. In the interim he had remained with his father. Agnes left her stepdaughter with learning disabilities at home and it was a constant worry to her to know what was happening; she felt guilty for leaving her and needed to know she was safe.

Housing needs

Under the 1990 NHS Community Care Act one of the fundamental principles is choice. Yet the range of choices offered to older women often seems limited. Even though the care management process is intended to be needs-led the system is still often very much resource-led. Thus, older women are usually offered the traditional resource of residential care, when in many cases other options should have been explored. Workers undertaking assessments are under constant pressure to assess quickly and in many abuse cases quick decisions are not appropriate. After living in the same situation for many years, making major life changes must be done at the victim's own pace, which may take a long time.

This was clearly illustrated in the case of Agnes, who wished to leave her husband after 30 years of marriage, because he had abused her physically, emotionally and financially. Agnes was assessed by an unqualified social worker and placed in a nursing home, where she did not settle at all. She was interviewed eight weeks after she had been placed there:

> "It was John [son] and Margaret [social worker] and the matron here that got me in here really and I didn't know for certain. I'd been around and I said, 'It looks a nice place', but I expected having a longer period to think about it and see other places. But all of a sudden John rings up from South Africa and says, 'Mum you've got a bed, you've got a room ... they want you in as soon as possible'. Well that put me in a panic. It was rushed, so therefore I think I'm still running I haven't put that brake on. I can't settle properly because I know there must be somewhere else where I would settle better ... well I have thought about sheltered accommodation." (Agnes)

Agnes moved from that nursing home to another and then eventually went into sheltered accommodation, where she is now happy and settled. Agnes had many doubts about how she would cope; she was scared about being on her own at night, and had not understood what could be available in a sheltered accommodation complex (for example, a warden on site, personal alarm system, home care support and so on). It is likely that had she been given more time to think early on in the process and been shown sheltered accommodation at the same time as the nursing home she would have been able to make the right choice at the beginning instead of having to make three moves.

Stella also felt that she was not part of the decision making:

> "I think at the bottom I am disappointed that I can't be part of it – people have seen it [the bungalow] and I haven't. I think I feel I am missing out." (Stella)

In child protection work a familiar question is: Why do we remove the children who have done nothing wrong and let the abuser stay at home? The same question is relevant to victims of elder abuse. The case of Catherine illustrates the need to consider this issue and also the need for solicitors and barristers with expertise in the field.

Catherine is 60 years old. She has had two brain tumours removed, which has left her with communication difficulties, epilepsy, partial sight and partial paralysis on the right side. Catherine was physically and financially abused by her son-in-law, who lived with her and her daughter, who had mental health problems. There was a joint tenancy in the names of Catherine and her daughter. She left the situation and moved temporarily to a resource centre. She wanted to return to her house, where she had lived happily with her husband (now deceased) for 35 years. A local solicitor was approached in order to apply to the court for a non-molestation order and occupation order. This solicitor did not have the expertise in this area of work and consequently did little to support Catherine's application to the court. On the other hand, the son-in-law's solicitor worked very hard to provide affidavits stating that Catherine was violent towards her son-in-law. Catherine had to go to court on three different occasions. Her solicitor did little to provide evidence that Catherine is not physically capable of being violent. No medical reports were prepared; her other daughters were not approached to make affidavits. Catherine lost her application and the occupation order was given to her daughter and son-in-law. Catherine was rehoused in another area.

In other cases, victims had been encouraged by family members to move from their homes where they had lived for many years. Some had been persuaded to move into "more suitable accommodation". This sometimes suited the needs of the carer rather than the victim, for example, the accommodation was closer and more convenient to the carer. However, the home is often extremely important, because of good memories associated with it; many of the women had been born and lived all their lives in the same house:

> "We had always lived in that house – my mother and dad had that house when they were married ... I didn't like leaving it. I didn't want to leave it and I stopped as long as I could." (Harriet)

> "They [her two daughters] decided that I lived too far away. They wanted me nearer. They got me this flat before I had seen it and flitted me.... I'm not happy in that if I could walk I wouldn't stay in this sheltered accommodation. It's nice and it's free – I have got my own furniture in but I haven't got my own front door. It means a lot to me having my own door, especially as I am now because I could go with myself to the door for a bit of fresh air, have a look at the outside world but as I am, no, I can't. But I can't have everything can I?" (Daphne)

Finally, once in a safe place the victim needs to be able to obtain possessions, which have been left behind. In most cases, it will be necessary for someone else to negotiate access and make the arrangements: victims may prefer not to face the abuser themselves.

Needs having left an abusive situation

After leaving an abusive situation, a victim will have further practical and emotional needs, which must be assessed and monitored. She is likely to face a gamut of emotions and self-questioning (for example, Have I done the right thing?, Will I survive?). There will be continuing practical matters to sort out; mention has already been made of housing and financial matters, and possibly the need for advice and support on legal issues. In short, workers should not presume that work with the victim will be reduced once she has left the situation; the intensity of need may continue for some time into the future. The primary concern, however, is that of personal safety.

To feel safe

Many abusers threaten that they will find out where the victims are and this remains a continuing anxiety for some victims. It is important that workers, in whatever setting, ensure that safety can be maintained to put the victim's mind at ease. Vera's bed in the hospital ward was opposite the door and she talked of her fear of seeing her husband walk into the hospital ward; she said, 'I looked at everybody's feet as they walked in the door and I dreaded seeing his white trainers'. Nursing staff moved Vera's bed next to the nurses' station, so that she felt safer and could easily get help if he did appear.

Practical resources are also needed such as alarm systems and, most importantly, the victim needs to know that someone will check her safety, for example, a warden calling in or a regular telephone call. The fear of seeing or having contact with the abuser can be ongoing and should not be underestimated.

Counselling and therapy

It is important to assess *when* a victim needs to talk specifically about the abuse and her feelings. Some will want to 'close down' for a while and contemplate what is happening to them; some may feel 'all talked out'. Counselling and therapy can be useful, but workers need to be careful not to rush in at an inappropriate stage in the victims' feelings. Victims may not be ready to face this until much further into the future, when careful assessment will be needed to identify the right type of counselling and therapy.

Current needs

The current needs of the victims interviewed frequently related to experiences in earlier life, to the abuse they had experienced more recently and to the relationship between these abusive experiences.

To talk

Although older women traditionally believe that personal matters should be kept to oneself, it is evident in both interviews and focus groups that victims of abuse do have a need to talk about their lives (past and present) and their abusive experiences. It is recognised that older people want to come to terms with past trauma in the later stages of life (certainly before they die), and many bring out unresolved issues or conflicts when they are approaching death (Hunt et al, 1997). It is true that some victims develop coping strategies, which may result in their forgetting or denying what has happened to them. Nonetheless, at some point the need to talk will usually arise. Sometimes, as noted earlier, it is easier to talk to a stranger, who has the necessary skills and sensitivity to provide a safe environment in which to talk openly and honestly. Indicating to a person that she has permission to talk and that she will be believed and not judged, can facilitate disclosure about abuse.

A sensitive balance needs to be found between seeking objectivity about factual circumstances (particularly when legal process may be involved) and accepting the victim's interpretation of those facts, and the 'truths' behind the memories – whether or not they appear to have been reconstructed in some situations.

When the findings of the project were fed back to victims in a focus group, the women readily started to share their stories with each other. They found it useful to listen to the experiences of others and Vera said it encouraged her to tell more. She said she had felt 'at ease' with the researcher, but felt that she could share even more with women who had gone through the same experiences as herself. This clearly indicated the need for peer group support.

The timing of the need to talk can vary for each individual. Some victims just need to tell the story once, in depth, and then they will 'want to forget'. Others may need to talk about the abuse regularly in order to work through anger and other unresolved issues. Some may say that they want to talk and then change their mind. During these interviews the women said that it was easier to talk to someone 'outside', that is, not the family or the worker(s) they saw regularly (for example, a social worker, day care workers, residential workers):

> "I was so ashamed that it was my own family had touched me; no I couldn't talk ... I couldn't discuss it. This is the first time I have discussed it from beginning to end but I am getting over it now." (Daphne)

Margaret told her story in full and then said at the end of the interview,

> "I don't want to remember it ... I don't want to talk about it. I want to put it out of my mind if I can. It's all in the past." (Margaret)

In some cases it was necessary to follow up the first interview, because the victim had 'not finished' or it was inappropriate to refer the victim on after the first interview. This was especially true in the case of Beatrice.

Beatrice is 91 years old. She attends day care twice a week and has regular respite care. For a long time she had said to staff in the centre, "I've had a terrible life. You wouldn't believe what happened to me". Staff had never pursued this but referred her to the researcher. Beatrice had been abused throughout her life by different people, but what she needed to talk about was the sexual abuse she had experienced from her brother. What she had never told anyone in her life was that she had become pregnant and the baby had died: "I had a baby when I was 16. It's true. I don't know how it happened. It lived, but there was nobody there to see it. It should have been in an incubator. It was a girl".

Beatrice did not want the staff in the centre to be told about the baby. She did not want to talk about the abuse or the baby again, but staff commented how Beatrice had changed since the first interview. They said she had become less agitated, more relaxed and happy.

During the in-depth interviews women were encouraged to talk about their lives from their earliest memory to the present day. Most enjoyed this, but were worried that they were 'boring'. (This reiterates the point that victims need to be given indicators that they have 'permission' to speak.) The use of reminiscence work is extremely important. All the women had experienced losses throughout their lives. Years ago morbidity rates were higher so that the loss of siblings and children was commonplace; even so there is still a need to talk about them. Other types of losses had not been addressed.

Hilda's children had been taken off her when they were very young and were brought up by their paternal grandmother. Hilda started hearing voices a year after she married. She had frequent admissions to hospital and took frequent drug overdoses. Hilda is physically and financially abused by her son, but has no contact with her daughter. She has only seen her "twice – at a funeral – she doesn't know who I am".

Isabella has mild learning disabilities, but years ago she was considered educationally subnormal. She became pregnant in her teens and was consequently committed to a mental institution for 20 years. She lost the baby and years of her life.

Another need was to talk about regrets, that is, about what they had not done or not achieved:

Stella is 89 years old and lives with her husband who she described as "one big problem". She felt she was being emotionally abused by her family and was very depressed. She had nightmares every night and sometimes in the day when she fell asleep. During the interview she realised that this had started when she had heard that a former boyfriend had died 12 months previously. She regretted not marrying him when she had the chance and had always known what he was doing during the past 70 years because he was a well-known local artist.

Bertha was very bitter about a number of things in her life:

"... there is no doubt my parents turned to me always ... if anything happened in the family and needed settling I was dragged into it.... We didn't have any babies unfortunately but we had plenty of kids in the family ... I have looked after all the kids in the family ... that is how it worked out – I was the available auntie ... the only drawback in my time was the fact that if you were a miner's daughter you didn't qualify for a good job." (Bertha)

Information
It has been shown that most victims of abuse choose to continue living in the abusive situation; this may be for a number of different reasons (Pritchard, 1995). However, a major reason is that maintaining a relationship with the abuser is more important than stopping the abuse. Therefore, the victim may need information about the abuser's own problem(s). Joan and Florence had lived in similar situations; both had brought up their grandsons, who were drug users and suppliers. Both young men physically and financially abused their grandmothers in order to finance their habits. Although information about drugs is widely available, often it is not circulated where older people have

access to it. This emphasises the need for dissemination of information in various forms to older people in the community. Although drug abuse was the main problem highlighted by women in this project, alcohol abuse is often a factor in elder abuse, and information about such problems is important.

Other useful practical information may be needed on various topics. For example, Catherine wanted to know what it would be like in a courtroom, and wanted help in preparing to make an application for a non-molestation order and occupation order (1996 Family Law Act).

Food and warmth

In the interviews and focus groups participants were asked to consider two things: What are your needs now?, What is most important to you now? Overwhelmingly, the responses were about food and warmth. In interviews most women talked at length about the poverty and hardship they had experienced. Gwen remembered as a child being sent in the mornings to the chip shop for cold scraps. Most of them had worked all of their lives in order to get food for themselves or their families:

> "I have had to bake to bring mine [the children] up." (Martha)

Beatrice talked about the conditions she had worked in when in service:

> "She had a wash-house outside. I would be washing in there and had icicles running down the windows. I didn't think anything about it. I was used to it. But it built me up because I got my food...." (Beatrice)

What was important to the women now was to be comfortable and not have to struggle anymore:

> "I have been so poor and so hard up. I have been very hungry at times, but I feel I have a lovely pension, about £140 a week. I feel like a millionaire. I have a new carpet down; that is happiness to me." (Beatrice)

When visiting day centres, service users were asked what they liked most about the centres and the responses were always about the warmth, the food and the companionship.

Company/social contact

One of the most crucial needs was to combat loneliness. Participants in the focus groups who attended day care facilities indicated that the main benefit was meeting other people. Victims often felt isolated in their homes and talked about the days being very long. However, workers need to find more imaginative ways to help combat loneliness and individual assessment is crucial – it should not be assumed that everyone enjoys the same activities or wants to be part of a group. Day care is frequently offered to people who want social contact but do not want to mix with other people in that setting. This highlights the needs for more individual, outreach work, in the community. Until some 30 years ago, many voluntary community organisations ran 'friendly visiting' schemes for the housebound, but such schemes no longer exist due to a lack of organisational funding; they do not fit the fashionable criteria of defined tasks, projected costs and provable benefits. However, Gwen welcomed the weekly visit from a volunteer, who had been requested by the GP in order to get Gwen to talk about her depression.

It should not be forgotten that victims placed in residential care can also feel isolated, because their previous social activities (for example, day care) have been stopped. Agnes felt very frustrated in the nursing home because she could not get out:

> "I do need somewhere where I can get out and about on my own and go to a shop. There's no shops here ... I like the country or even gardens, trees and birds ands flowers ... I haven't been anywhere while I have been in here eight weeks." (Agnes)

In contrast, Georgina had been placed in a home which organised weekly outings (for pub lunches, shopping trips to large shopping centres and so on) and other social activities, which actually improved Georgina's quality of life. Life had also improved for Joan and Isabella, who had moved to sheltered accommodation where wardens organised social events on a daily basis. Isabella and her co-tenants were provided with lunch and eating times were seen as important in bringing people together.

> ## To summarise, victims said that they needed to:
>
> - meet people
> - go shopping
> - have social outings
> - have holidays
> - revisit favourite places

Hobbies and interests

For many victims it was also important to remain occupied and keep previous hobbies and interests. This was another area which was seldom adequately assessed. Workers spent little time finding out about the interests (past and present) of those they were helping. Daphne, who has had one leg amputated, enjoys craftwork:

> "I look forward to Fridays, but I am wanting to come on Mondays as it is art and craft day and I do a lot of beadwork, making necklaces ... I know I could knock on with it here because there is tables and everything ... and if I have to do it in a chair the beads are rolling all over so." (Daphne)

Victims also mentioned the types of novels they enjoyed reading, the television programmes they watched regularly, the types of videos they wanted to see and other things they enjoyed (knitting, crocheting, sewing). These things were a very important part of their daily lives.

Religion

Religion is important to many older people and continues to be a great help to them: "I believe in God and he helps me" (Beatrice).

Again this need is often neglected, perhaps because religion is less important to many younger people. It is essential that victims are able to follow their beliefs and that their spiritual needs are supported, for example, it was important to Georgina that the priest visited her every week in the residential home to give her communion. Sometimes belief in God has helped them survive in the abusive situation and to adapt to a new environment.

Health and hygiene

When undertaking a 'full needs' assessment, one would assume the importance of health matters; however, it was apparent in the project that some professionals had ignored the health needs of the victims. Furthermore, some workers were not aware (because of lack of training) of the long-term effects of certain types of abuse (for example, permanent internal damage, chronic eating disorders, self-harm/self-neglect, suicidal tendencies and nightmares or flashbacks).

When victims have experienced violence, there can be permanent physical and mental damage. Vera had had 10 pregnancies; only two children survived. The violence she experienced from her husband (hitting and kicking in the stomach) caused the miscarriages and death of her babies.

Lilian believed many of her current health problems were a direct result of the physical violence she had experienced from her husband:

> "I have a funny throat because he tried to choke me one time and it keeps coming, this peculiar throat. They found out in hospital that I had a malfunctioning kidney. Well that could have been with the thumps." (Lillian)

> "[My brother] was rotten ... I think he is the cause of my deafness. Bashing me or running at you with a kick ... he used to kick me to the ground.... I have been hit too much." (Beatrice)

Often, inadequate time had been spent with victims to assess their current health problems. In interview with Hilda, who suffers with schizophrenia, I was concerned about her low weight and the severe soreness of her eyes, which were obviously causing her great discomfort. I contacted the social worker to voice my concerns. When I had asked Hilda about her health problems she was resigned to the fact that she had to take medication (largactil) – "I have been taking them for 30 years" – and felt nothing could be done about her other physical ailments. Hilda has numerous medical problems including partial sight, arthritis in her knees, an over active thyroid; she has a long history of drug overdoses and self-neglect.

It is a matter of concern that health needs are often not assessed properly either in the community or in residential settings:

> Gertrude is 92 and was placed in a nursing home six months ago. She has been financially abused by a neighbour. Gertrude has a tumour in her breast; it is thought that she will live for some time yet. She is extremely deaf. No one has done anything about her hearing problem.

Martha had been visited by the practice nurse the day before her interview and she was worried about a number of things. The nurse had not explained why she was taking blood from her and Martha wondered why she no longer got thyroxin tablets from her GP. She had not felt able to ask the nurse about this. This emphasises the need for time to be spent with older women to give them clear explanations and to ensure that they are not left worrying about their health and medical conditions.

The body is particularly important to victims who have been sexually abused. Workers need to be sensitive to the fact that some victims may not wish to be touched at all; even a slight touch on the arm may trigger a flashback. Also, having to be clean can become an obsession, and hygiene can be extremely important to a victim.

To reduce the fear of crime

Police say that the fear of crime is far greater than its prevalence. However, there were a large number of people in focus groups who had been victims of crime – mainly burglaries or muggings in the street; five women interviewed (Beatrice, Georgina, Jessie, Martha and Rose) had been victims of physical and financial abuse by strangers. Previous work on gang abuse (Pritchard, 1993, 1995) was reinforced by this project's findings. In all three areas where this project took place, older people were being targeted by gangs of young children or youths.

"Well last time there were lads, about 20 and they were big. I just don't say anything. They do it all the more. Two or three nights there were about 20 of them." (Rose)

The most vulnerable people were those living in sheltered accommodation complexes or in quiet areas, where there were large populations of older people:

"They have been more than twice in here.... That lad has just come out of prison not long since ... I think he has had to do about five or six month.... It's as though you have been raped in a way, coming into your house. Terrible. An awful feeling." (Martha)

It was generally felt that the police did not take the matter seriously and did not respond quickly when called:

"A community policeman came and another one came. I said, 'Are you looking for clues?'. He said, 'No, I have lost a button from my uniform'." (Rose)

"It's crime prevention they always focus on. Burglaries and things [pause]. But the muggings bit they don't seem to be interested." (Jessie)

There was general concern about having only one telephone number for the police (most forces now have a central number to cover a wide area). Older people said they would like to have local numbers and to be able to get in touch with local police stations directly. Participants in the focus groups were very clear that they would like to see the return of community police in their areas, visibly patrolling the streets. Victims felt safer when they knew they had people close to them (for example, a warden), some sort of alarm system, or, as in some areas, close circuit television cameras had been installed.

Summary: The key needs identified are:

Advice	Religion
Choice/options	Trust
Company	To get out and about
Control over own life/own affairs	To talk
Counselling	To stop the abuse/violence
Food and warmth	To leave the abusive situation
Health	To be safe
Hobbies/interests	To be believed
Housing	To be listened to
Information	To protect family/abuser
Money/benefits/pension	To forget about what has happened
People	To reduce fear of crime
Physical help	To feel safe in the house/community
Place of safety	To know who to go to for help
Practical help	To have telephone numbers
Privacy	

6

Needs from the workers' perspectives

Towards the end of the project every worker who had completed a monitoring form in the past two years was invited to attend a focus group in order to discuss the needs of elder abuse victims. The 40 workers who attended included:

- team managers of fieldwork teams;
- managers of residential units;
- social workers from area offices and hospital-based teams;
- unqualified social workers/assessors;
- home care organisers;
- a Diploma in Social Work student on placement.

Focus groups were run in each department – two in Churchtown because of high interest. The advertised aim was to see which needs were identified by workers and to make comparisons with the needs as identified by victims. At the beginning of the session members were given 10 minutes preparation time to think about the topic of the needs of elder abuse victims and were asked to make notes. The sessions ran for two hours. At the end of each group the main findings from the project were fed back. The aim of this chapter is to present the key points from the discussions.

The subject areas which arose in the discussions were similar in each of the four groups. The only main difference to be observed was in the amount of detail given by workers from Churchtown, who expressed greater clarity about what was needed by victims. It was particularly interesting that, although groups began by talking about victims' needs – the words 'safety' and 'protection' were mentioned immediately – the discussion quickly drifted into the difficulties and frustrations felt by the workers in working with problems of elder abuse. We were, almost at once, addressing the needs of the workers rather than those of the victims. It was clear that workers welcomed the opportunity to talk to each other about the difficulties they experienced. Discussions focused on problems in working with victims (for example, victims wanting to remain in the abusive situation), difficulties within each department (for example, lack of time and resources), lack of support from managers and the specific demands of individual cases.

Understanding elder abuse

In all the groups there were predominantly negative attitudes to this area of work, particularly that little can be done because:

- victims may not recognise the situation as abusive – it is 'normal' for them;
- victims usually do not want any intervention;
- there is no legislative framework as there is in child protection work.

> "In an abusive situation for a long period of time they don't identify it as abuse. It's their way of life. Although they may not be comfortable with it, they may not be happy about it, they just see it as the way it is." (Worker, Tallyborough)

> "We have no legislation, whereas in childcare you have got the various acts where you can take someone into care. We cannot do that as we have no legislation and that makes our work even more difficult really, when you know abuse is going on you just cannot do anything." (Worker, Tallyborough)

Some workers who attended were very experienced and there appeared to be a trend within the departments for the same workers to pick up the elder abuse cases. However, the fundamental problem is that many workers do not have enough knowledge or understanding about the whole issue of elder abuse; especially in the identification of abuse and the long-term effects of abuse on the victim. This results in a belief that little can be done to help victims. It was evident that the majority of workers wanted to 'rescue' victims from the abusive situation rather than to work with them while remaining in the situation. There needs to be a fundamental shift in ways of thinking and working with victims.

Lack of knowledge results in a lack of confidence when involved in an investigation or when monitoring a situation in the long term. This highlights the need for intensive and regular training, and also for the development of specialisation for both workers (in all settings) and managers. Workers often felt unsupported because managers did not have sufficient knowledge in this area of work, and so were unable to advise and support the worker adequately. Workers in Churchtown talked specifically about needing to understand more about why abuse happens, the cycle of abuse and understanding the motives of perpetrators.

Particular training needs are:

- Definition of abuse
- Signs and symptoms
- How to investigate
- Interviewing skills
- Understanding why abuse happens
- Understanding abusers

Time pressures

Workers felt under pressure to get things done quickly, so that investigations were often rushed. Also, because of the number of general referrals, cases were sometimes closed when they should have been kept open for monitoring purposes:

> "We all want a quick fix. Including the care managers." (Worker, Tallyborough)

> "We go through work like the speed of sound." (Worker, Millfield)

> "I'm a firm believer in prevention rather than intervention and it is our department that stopped all the preventative work and the long-term cases where you went every week to visit and it was 'get the kettle on', which has all gone and I disagree with." (Worker, Churchtown)

The overall conclusion in all the groups was that there was not enough time to do the 'ordinary' (in other words, statutory) work, never mind elder abuse work, and it is consequently not given enough priority.

In Tallyborough's focus group, there was a long discussion about how assessments are undertaken and all the administrative work which has to be done.

> **Worker A:** "What we tend to end up doing, I think, is fulfilling all the administrative functions of an assessment with the forms that we have to fill in and who we have to send them to, and in a way the priority should be the client but it isn't. We are forced into filling all these forms in to justify what we are doing and they overtake the needs of the client that we are dealing with."

> **Worker B:** "I agree. That's one of the things I have written down here that the actual victim that I was dealing with at that particular time I didn't spend enough time with her. I know I didn't because of other commitments."

> **Worker C:** "We are discouraged generally from actually spending a lot of time. The focus is always on doing your assessment and filling out the forms and putting in the practical, and we don't really look at emotional needs."

Ethical issues

Discussions also focused on professional dilemmas – in particular ethical issues around breaking confidentiality. It was said that sometimes decisions are taken away from the victim, for example, when informing the police that a crime has taken place, and this conflicts with basic social work values and the victim's civil rights. Some workers felt that the local police were not helpful when dealing with elder abuse referrals (this was especially true in Millfield) and that GPs' general lack of awareness about abuse did not help. At other times, workers felt they colluded with the victim by not telling and by taking no further action, because the victim wished to stay in the abusive situation.

Another concern was that when there are investigations into abuse by residential or day care staff, the needs of the victim are often ignored. This led to comments about the fact that, even when workers identify needs, there are insufficient resources to draw upon. This exacerbates the individual worker's sense of isolation – in which there is inadequate partnership with other services, inadequate training and supervision, very low priority, and virtually no legislated duties. Work with older victims becomes almost entirely an individual professional decision in competition with more formal duties.

In Tallyborough, workers felt strongly that the resources available were often inappropriate and services too inflexible to suit the needs of victims. They suggested that there needed to be more emphasis on working with victims in their own homes (outreach work) rather than sending victims to the 'usual resources like day care'.

The air of despondency found in all the focus groups is another cause for concern. If negative attitudes prevail, it is unlikely that workers are going to work in an imaginative way; this was validated when the findings of the project were fed back to the workers, which is discussed below.

Inter-agency working

A common theme in all groups was problems in liaising with other agencies. The police were often the main target for criticism:

> "I found the nursing staff took the abuse seriously. When they actually contacted the police, they didn't. They came to a meeting on the ward but they weren't interested in what the person had to say." (Worker, Churchtown)

> "I have used the police in the past but what generally happens is they come back and say you need to substantiate the evidence and you can't gather enough to prove it." (Worker, Tallyborough).

Other problems included working with other professionals (for example, within hospitals) who "lack understanding" and "tell us what to do":

> "I felt that while it was being investigated there should have been somewhere where she could go to be counselled to talk it through and even on the ward it was quite [pause] ... I found it oppressive. It wasn't a nice relaxed atmosphere. Things had to be done at a rate and not at her time because they wanted her out of hospital." (Worker, Churchtown)

"I had a run in with professionals on my ward. I am sat with a guy ... he's 92 and he wants to go home and your physio team is saying he has got to do all these things and I got really cross because they weren't talking to this man. They were talking to me. So I let it go for about half an hour and he just cried. I said, 'Do you realise that man is 92 years old? He has lived at home without his wife for 30 years and you are telling him how to walk and how to go to the toilet and when to eat...'. They said, 'He's got to listen'.... They weren't giving him a choice." (Worker, Churchtown)

Workers' perspectives of victims' needs

When discussion did focus on the needs of the victim, it was evident that ideas and comments essentially emanated from the format of the assessment procedures drawn up by departments under the 1990 NHS and Community Care Act. If we look back at the needs identified by victims in Chapter 5, it is clear that they were much more specific. This again confirms the point that workers may not be undertaking assessments in an holistic way. For example, there was little recognition of the importance of leisure activities, interests, hobbies and education to an older person. When talking about needs, workers tended predominantly to use social work jargon couched in very global and general terms, as can be seen below. This was particularly so in Tallyborough and Millfield; workers in Churchtown were much more specific about actual and precise needs:

"There is a need for pro-active services." (Worker, Millfield)

"To establish some trust and confidence." (Worker, Tallyborough)

There was a marked contrast in the ways in which needs were defined and described by workers and by victims – the latter found it easy to explain what their needs were. Thus, for example, workers talked about needing *information*, but this was mainly in relation to their own needs rather than those of the victims. No reference was made to the specific information and advice itemised by victims (see the summary on page 74). This begs the question whether workers and victims have different perspectives and whether there is a common understanding.

Victims' needs, as identified by the workers, and the common needs which were identified by both victims and workers (shown in bold) are as follows:

- Access to help 24 hours a day
- Anger management
- Appropriate setting to disclose/talk about abuse
- Awareness that situation is abusive
- Be understood
- Build self-esteem
- **Choice/options/alternatives**
- Confidentiality
- Consistency in worker(s)
- Draw strength from other victims
- Easy access to services
- Emotional needs/support
- Empathy
- Maintain confidentiality
- **Maintain relationships (for example, with abuser; same worker)**
- **Place of safety**
- Preventative work
- **Privacy**
- Protection
- Reduce anxiety
- **Safety/security**
- Safety to disclose
- **Social contacts/outlets**
- Someone to manage/deal with finances
- Someone to support victim during investigation interview
- Specialist resources
- Sympathy
- To be assertive
- **To be in control**
- **To be taken seriously**
- To feel comfortable with worker(s) undertaking investigations
- To feel confident
- To see that life could be different
- **To talk**
- **Trust**

All the groups identified the victim's need to talk, but again highlighted the problem of finding adequate time to do this:

> "She'd got all the services in place but for me to discuss what was happening to her and how she was feeling about the situation – I just didn't have the time to do that." (Worker, Tallyborough)

> "We need a body of workers to go and sit for a few hours. Social workers haven't got the time." (Worker, Millfield)

Availability of workers was thought to be crucial, especially as crises (the abuse) tend to happen at night. Workers in Millfield and Churchtown felt there should be workers available to respond 24 hours a day.

Workers in Churchtown talked at length about what should be available when a victim decides to leave her situation, what the new environment should be like and the importance of not relying on the usual 'institutions'.

> "A homely environment, perhaps not a residential home, possibly something not institutionalised. Something homely like somebody's home with no uniforms on. Just very informal and do it at their pace. Where they have a lounge, a kitchen and a bathroom." (Worker, Churchtown)

> "I think there should be emotional literacy courses especially for the family because they all can't see that there is a problem but there obviously is so they all need to be counselled." (Worker, Churchtown)

Problems working with abusers

All groups talked about the difficulties in working with abusers, especially in cases where the abuse is by family members and carers. Workers from Millfield spoke at length about financial abuse and the need for specialist advice (to workers in particular regarding the legal situation) and to manage the victim's finances. In Tallyborough and Millfield workers talked about the difficulty of working with cases where family members are financially abusing a dependent victim by taking their benefits: "We are toothless tigers" (Worker, Millfield).

Needs from the workers' perspectives

These two groups also talked about the needs of abusive carers. It was felt that carers are often pushed into the caring role and may lack the skills and practical information they need:

> "Some people's capacity to care is limited and that needs to be recognised. Some are good carers and do it naturally, others have not got the capacity to care and I think it is important for the worker to recognise that." (Worker, Tallyborough)

It was also felt that many abusive situations could be prevented if carers had access to more resources:

> "Prevention – that's one thing we don't do. We investigate and don't look at prevention." (Worker, Millfield)

The key needs of carers can be summarised as:

- To be paid a living wage
- Education and training – how to care; recognition of abuse
- Supervision and management
- Information and to provide appropriate resources
- Support (from workers and group support)
- To relieve pressures and tensions of caring
- Social outlets

As mentioned above, workers in Churchtown focused on the need to know why someone abuses, but they also discussed the fact that victims can be difficult to work with because they have particular needs. Examples were given of cases where the victim needed 'to control', 'to control the family', 'be manipulative', 'be abused'.

Workers' views of victims' opinions

At the end of each session the needs expressed by victims were presented. Workers found the findings surprising in regard to:

- the detail of need as specified by victims;
- the long-term effect of abuse (for example, eating disorders, behaviour traits, flashbacks, the importance of the body and the need for hygiene);
- wish to involve police (one worker admitted "Maybe if I am honest, I have never asked a victim if they want the police involved. Maybe it's my own prejudices");
- victims wanting to leave abusive situations when they are older;
- victims requesting precise information;
- victims stating that they had wanted someone to ask them if they were being abused.

What was clear was that workers generally may not have an understanding of whether a victim wants to leave an abusive situation or remain in it. Workers may need to make connections between the needs of younger and older victims of abuse. There needs to be a firm foundation for understanding the short- and long-term effects of abuse. Workers who have worked in the child protection field may make some connections, but the majority of workers in the adult sector may never have had training on this subject. Also, workers need to be aware that older women will seek similar information and advice to a younger victim with regard to money, housing, the law and so on. It appears that workers may be working in oppressive ways that see older women as 'different' and resistant to change, whereas the women interviewed in this project clearly welcomed change.

Summary: The key needs of workers are:

Professional needs

Competence in the definition of abuse; how to recognise abuse; confidence in working with victims and in investigating; more time to work with victim; time to do investigation properly/thoroughly; time to sit and think; go at victim's pace, not to the department's time-scales; risk assessments; skills – empowerment, assertiveness, enabling, confrontation; elder abuse cases should not be closed due to other pressures.

Support and supervision

Clear guidelines for action; consistency within the social services department; support from managers and the department; give time to emotional feelings of workers; recognition that some workers cannot work with elder abuse; training.

Specialisation of tasks

Specialist teams; two workers – one for victim, one for abuser.

Legislative framework

Power to take decision away from victim; police to take referrals seriously; access to legal advice.

Inter-agency working

Communication; sharing of information.

7

Services and resources: good practice recommendations

Over the last decade there has been general agreement that work with elder abuse should be done in a multi-disciplinary way. As policies have developed, there has been an emphasis on an inter-agency approach. The findings from this research project confirm that, first, practical help and support are needed from workers in a wide range of agencies and, second, the resources required are not always offered or are not readily available to older victims. This chapter makes good practice suggestions for agencies and workers who might be able to provide for the needs of older women. The findings presented in this chapter have been discussed with, and validated by, a number of the original interviewees.

Confronting ageism

Ageism needs to be confronted to provide older victims with the appropriate resources. Resources offered to younger victims are not automatically offered to older women (for example, rape counselling). There may be a number of reasons for this, but managers should ensure that workers in all settings are not discriminatory in their practice. It is clear that older women may decide to leave an abusive situation, even when they have lived in that situation for a large part of their lives and it should not be presumed that they are not capable of change. Many established organisations could offer help to older women, provided they accommodate any special requirements, such as, transport for those with mobility problems.

Publicity

It is often very difficult for victims of abuse to talk about what they have experienced and to ask for help; also, elder abuse is still largely a taboo subject and the general public is unaware of its prevalence. The issue of elder abuse needs to be given a higher profile and organisations need to advertise the fact that they are available to help older victims.

Media campaigns and presence in television programmes have made the public more aware of problems such as domestic violence, and similar action is needed regarding elder abuse. Older women may not know where to turn and therefore posters and leaflets are needed to publicise what help is available, and to provide local contact numbers and addresses. This is discussed further below. Different media need to be used to circulate this information as many victims remain hidden and isolated because they are not known to any agency. It should also be remembered that a number of older people are illiterate.

Good methods of creating awareness are:

- Leaflets/posters (distributed in places where older people visit)
- Local and national newspapers
- Radio and television
- Information centres/mobile buses
- Insertions in utility bills

Resources in the short and long term

Current practices indicate that there is emphasis on completing short-term work, but not enough time spent on considering provision of resources in the long term, even though taking a longer view is a requirement of the care management process. In elder abuse work, there may be a lot of activity among workers in different agencies during the course of an abuse investigation. Investigation should include an assessment of risk, which is presented at a case conference, and from this a protection plan should be developed to provide appropriate resources in the long term (Pritchard, 1999). However, the present climate of budget cuts and limited resources has the damaging effect of discouraging workers from thinking creatively for the long term. There may be resources which could meet the long-term needs of victims as mentioned in Chapters 5 and 6.

Resource files

Teams of workers should develop a resource file of useful resources and in what ways they were found to be helpful. Some workers deal with elder abuse cases infrequently and may forget useful contacts for the next time unless recorded.

Key information to note is:

- Name of person/organisation
- Address
- Telephone, fax numbers, email address
- Work specialism
- Why they were helpful

People and organisations who might be able to help

As this study shows, many types of workers could be the recipients of disclosure of elder abuse and may be asked by the victim for help.

The people cited by the interviewees as those who could give practical help and support are:

- Doctor in hospital
- Psychologist
- Psychiatrist
- GP
- Nurse – hospital and in the community
- Counsellor/therapist
- Citizens' Advice Bureau
- Department of Social Security
- Housing department/housing officer/housing associations
- Police – domestic violence officers/CID/community police officer
- Victim support
- Social services/social worker
- Solicitor
- Volunteer
- Visitor/befriender
- Advocate
- Workers in day centres/residential homes
- Vicar/priest etc

Every victim of elder abuse will have individual needs, and it is therefore impossible to generalise who the most appropriate person to talk to will be. Trust and building confidence are very important, although a victim may find it easier to tell a stranger what has happened to her rather than someone she knows well. This was true of Joan, who found it easier to tell the psychiatrist in hospital about her grandson abusing her rather than disclosing to her social worker, whom she had known for a long time:

> "I have a psychiatrist specialist to talk to me and social services have come a lot to try and get it out of me. You see I wouldn't say anything, I kept everything to myself.... They were a long time before they got anything out of me." (Joan)

Workers in medical settings (such as nurses and doctors in hospitals, GP practices and community nurses) are likely to be the people who hear disclosure at a time of crisis. In the focus group, both Vera and Joan said they that had found it particularly useful to have an allocated personal nurse on the ward when they were admitted to hospital. Other professionals who work within these settings could also have a role to play. Emma told her acupuncturist in the GP surgery what was happening to her: "She gave me encouragement. She explained to me that these days it is a crime". Other health workers approached included a physiotherapist, an occupational therapist, a speech therapist and a dietician.

Women often talk when a personal and intimate activity is taking place, for example, care staff in day care and residential settings may hear a disclosure when bathing or dressing someone.

Investigation and assessment

Following disclosure, it is crucial that consideration is given to who are the most appropriate people to undertake an investigation. Most departmental policies recommend that it should be a qualified social worker plus one other person. It appears to be of paramount importance that at least one of the investigating officers should be someone the victim knows and feels comfortable with, for example, the person to whom the abuse was initially disclosed, or some other trusted worker or advocate. The investigating officer's objective is to find out whether the victim has been abused and to assess the degree of risk for the future; especially if the victim wishes to continue living in the abusive situation. Consequently, the investigation involves a comprehensive assessment, which will identify the needs of the victim both immediately and in the longer term.

It is important during the short-term work that all necessary assessments are undertaken, for example, the victim may have injuries and require medical attention. It must be remembered that there is no legal provision to enforce a medical examination; nevertheless, consideration should be given to whether a full medical examination would be helpful if the victim has health problems. Workers must also be aware of the possible long-term effects of physical abuse, such as internal damage, eating disorders and so on. Also, if there are concerns about the victim's mental state, an assessment of capacity should be undertaken, to be presented at the case conference. Thorough assessments may be needed to develop an appropriate protection plan; assessments should not be rushed simply to fit into the time-scales suggested in some elder abuse policies.

There are other people who may also have a role to play during the abuse investigation. If the victim has communication difficulties, therapists could be brought in to help, such as communication, art or music therapists. Aromatherapists can be invaluable in helping the victim to relax both to facilitate disclosure, and in subsequent short- and long-term work. Before going to court Catherine could not sleep and was very anxious; the resource centre organised an aromatherapist to give Catherine a massage once a week and she was encouraged to use aromatherapy oils on a daily basis, all of which had a positive effect.

Legal advice

One of the women's most important needs was for practical advice about legal matters. Specialist solicitors need to be available to give advice (both to workers and victims) regarding divorce, dealing with harassment and violence, and the management of finances. It is important that social workers find local specialists in different aspects of the law. As can be seen in the case of Catherine, instructing a solicitor who lacks expertise in the particular field required can have devastating effects. Legal advice can be available through Citizens' Advice Bureaux and Law Centres, who may hold regular surgeries. These surgeries should be advertised and there needs to be information about costs and the criteria for applying for legal aid. What is also important to victims is contact with the solicitor in order to build trust and confidence:

> "She keeps constantly in touch with me either by letter or by 'phone of anything that needs to be done and, like I said, the money wasn't the important issue for me but the solicitor told me that if I didn't accept it then it was myself that I was harming because I had the right to half of whatever he had and he had hoarded this money from 1985 ... £30,256." (Vera)

Police

The police can have a crucial role to play and police forces need to be proactive in designating officers to deal with elder abuse. In Churchtown, victims said that the local domestic violence officer was extremely helpful and understanding. It is important that victims are talked to in a way that is neither patronising nor demeaning and does not use jargon, in addition to the provision of practical resources to make them feel safe.

> "He [domestic violence officer] is very open in the way he speaks to people. I found that he understood the position I was in so therefore he knew the help I needed from him. He knew that I was nervous and I was afraid so to make me feel that much more comfortable he decided to put the police alarm in. I have a button I wear round my neck and it just needs the slightest touch and the whole thing goes off." (Vera)

In the other two departments victims were more critical of the police, especially with regard to crime in the community and slow response times. In Tallyborough, Jessie commented:

> "I have now got one of these personal alarms. If I pull that it will make a terrible noise. There should be more of these handed out and more contact numbers." (Jessie)

Police forces also need to be clear that different officers are needed to address different situations. A domestic violence officer has a role in advising and helping a victim to leave an abusive situation, while community police will also be needed by older victims of crime within the community:

> "They [police] don't seem interested. On this estate we are vulnerable because we have only got wardens. The police don't protect or come round here. There should be community police on this estate. Once we had a policeman. He got killed in a car and we have never had a community policeman since and I live on the ground floor which is next to here, and you can see the centre and kids always smashing the centre up. I have called the police no end of times." (Jessie)

> "A community policeman came and another one came.... It's just to feel that someone is bothered." (Rose)

Another criticism which emerged from both interviews and focus groups was that when the police are contacted the response is often slow and it sometimes takes hours for them to arrive. It was felt that patrol cars should be able to respond immediately, but this did not happen because harassment in certain localities is not taken seriously when it happens on a regular basis.

The police sometimes refer victims to Victim Support and this was often helpful:

> "Well I have got £90 back off that lad, but there will have been more than that taken. I have had someone down from Victim Support and she helped me write it all down.... She [volunteer from Victim Support] knew how to help." (Martha)

However, not all victims had been referred to Victim Support, despite its potential usefulness. Jessie was mugged in the street and would have welcomed contact from Victim Support "but it wasn't even mentioned".

A regular comment from women in the focus groups was that they were unsure who to contact and did not like having one central number for the police which covered a wide geographical area. One woman reported that the local newspaper had printed a list of useful emergency numbers for older people; she had cut this out and pinned it on her kitchen wall (in a clear polythene bag) for future use. This is an idea which should be developed by all agencies, so that victims are clear about who to contact and have telephone numbers which are up to date. The idea of helplines was welcomed in interviews and focus groups, but again women said that contact numbers would have to be widely advertised – most of them had no idea how to contact the local helplines which were already available.

Benefits and finances

Anxieties about benefits and financial matters were common among victims who had left abusive situations. They stressed that they needed information before leaving, but that, in most cases, these issues had been sorted out afterwards. It often it took a long time (up to three months in some cases) to sort out their entitlements, which added to the victims' worries: they did not like "owing money to anyone". The benefits system is complex and victims suggested that simple explanations should be available and that DSS officers need to be able to visit people quickly to advise and help them with the completion of forms. When interviewed, Joan was still trying to sort out her financial situation after moving into sheltered accommodation; the situation was complicated by the fact that her husband was living in a nursing home:

> "I wrote and told them. They don't take any notice. They just ignore it. So now I have a load of things to send to Newcastle because they are stopping his money until they get it." (Joan)

Victims had little knowledge about:

- benefits in general, that is, what they were entitled to apply for;
- housing benefit and how that fits in with the payment of rent;
- additional payments, for example, to help with purchasing essential items, furniture, decorating.

In some cases, it was only after DSS officers had visited that victims realised they were entitled to additional benefits because of disability. They said that had they known this before it would have "saved a lot of worrying for nothing".

A 'link person'

During the focus group, victims said that once they had left the abusive situation they often had to repeat their story to a number of officials from different agencies. They suggested having a 'link person' to assess their needs and coordinate the responses; the social worker was thought to be the best person to do this.

It is also important for victims to have other practical matters sorted out at an early stage:

- Retrieving possessions/clothing from previous home
- Buying new clothes to replace clothing left behind
- Obtaining furniture

It was suggested that the link person could coordinate this and volunteers could be used to undertake some of the tasks. It was important for victims to be able to make their new home comfortable and some had received help from workers and neighbours:

"She [niece] has been absolutely wonderful to me. She has done all this ... made the curtains and the bedding and everything is her choice. She has thought of everything. After one day in the bedroom I thought I shall have to have a chair to sit on – I can't get my tights on. Next time she came she had got this chair for me – it's just the job." (Emma)

"I bought [from previous home] one wall unit, two chairs, one table which is behind the door, clothes dryer and the unit I have in the hallway.... This suite was given to me by a nurse from the ward I was on ... Social Security Fund they gave me £1,066. From that I got the carpet, the rug was thrown in free, pans, a cooker, fridge, a bed, wardrobe and a chest of drawers, and lino in the bathroom and in the kitchen. So they have done so much for me and it has left me feeling guilty because I have always had to beg for anything I wanted from him [husband] which was always turned down." (Vera)

Accommodation

A priority was having somewhere to live – initially a place of safety and eventually a permanent residence.

The victims said the following accommodation should be accessible:

- Hospital
- Council housing
- Refuges for older people
- Resource centres
- Safe houses
- Sheltered accommodation (with warden living on site)
- Older people's homes
- Private nursing homes

Timing is important – once a woman has decided to leave an abusive situation, she needs to know where she can go in order to plan her escape. An obstacle in the past has been that alternative accommodation was often not available for women and children. Local authority housing departments have a legal responsibility to rehouse victims living in domestic violence situations (1996 Housing Act), but many older people are unaware of this. Housing associations can also offer accommodation and it is important that workers have good links with these organisations and that housing officers are included in elder abuse investigations. Vera had found the local housing department particularly helpful when they attended a case conference:

"Without them I wouldn't have got this far, because they were with me all the way down the line, and they got me a council bungalow, and they got me all the security I needed, and they worked together." (Vera)

Vera was offered the bungalow 10 days after the case conference while she was still in hospital, but it is important that victims are not left wondering what is going to happen.

Not all women plan their escape; sometimes crises occur and emergency placements are required immediately. In Churchtown the resource centres provide very well for these situations, but this was not always the case in the other two departments where sometimes it was necessary for the victim to wait until a bed was found; in some cases this had been days or even weeks.

It may be older women's worst fear that they "will end up in an older people's home". It is necessary to consider alternative types of accommodation such as safe houses for older women. Local authorities could investigate housing options available for such situations. A refuge for older women was also suggested and this was considered more acceptable than "going into a home".

Thorough assessment of appropriate housing need is required. This project has found that some victims were placed in permanent residential care quickly, when, in fact, they may have been able to live in supported accommodation (see, for example, the discussion of Agnes' case in Chapter 5). Even though the 1990 NHS and Community Care Act promotes the concept of care in the community, it seems that many social workers are still too quick to consider permanent care as a suitable resource. It has been stressed previously that victims feel it is important to take control of their lives and most wish to remain as independent as possible.

Sheltered accommodation can be an excellent resource because such complexes provide:

- Safety
- Warden on site
- Company and contact with other residents
- Social activities

Ongoing support – the long-term work

Counselling and therapy

Victims may need to talk about their life and abusive experiences, but the timing of this will differ for individual victims:

> "I have reached the stage where I like to talk about it.... It doesn't make things better, but it makes you feel better." (Agnes)

There are many different forms of counselling and therapy and it is important that the most appropriate method is sought for each individual. Vera's social worker made a contract with her after she left hospital to continue seeing her on a weekly basis to provide counselling:

> "I have always been a good listener ... I was always ready to listen but then I wanted people to listen to me for once. There was so much bottled up inside and it was really tearing me apart.... It [counselling] has helped in the way that I haven't been holding on to some of the things that I needed to be rid of. We had talked in some depth but I still felt we weren't getting deeper enough into the problem and I think I know she herself thinks this – that there is a lot more talking to do." (Vera)

Some victims know they need to deal with their feelings but just do not know what could help them:

> "I can't believe that I have let this happen to me. I don't know how to get rid of the feeling of frustration and anger that I have allowed for someone to do that to me for 35 years. Because at the end of the day I don't want to be a victim. I want to be responsible for me and I feel why have I let that happen." (Mary)

When thinking about long-term help consideration must be given to the following factors:

- Specific problem(s) to be addressed
- Underpinning philosophy of helper
- Experience and understanding of elder abuse
- Methods to be used
- Gender of helper
- Age of helper
- Frequency of contact
- Appropriate venue for sessions (some victims may be housebound, others may still be living in abusive situations)

Victims made specific comments about what they thought was important in a helper:

> "It comes from people who have experienced it ... not being funny but half the time people don't understand what you go through until you have experienced it. I think you have no right to say anything. We have got a right but you don't want to say to them because you don't know how they are feeling. Such as me or anybody else we know exactly what is going on and we can feel for them and point them in the right direction." (Jessie)

> "I think a bit older person like myself. I think they would trust more than younger people." (Margaret)

> "My doctor is a woman and I think that makes a difference." (Mary)

Resources for long-term work
Resources need to be available to undertake effective long-term work with victims and this work could be undertaken in a number of centre settings.

Centres that could be used for monitoring and long-term work are:

- Day centres
- Day hospitals
- Community centres
- Women's centres
- Trauma centres

As indicated earlier, older women can benefit from resources usually associated with younger women.

Women's centres can offer a range activities:

- Social events
- Support groups
- Counselling
- Advice
- Courses – to develop specific skills such as assertiveness and empowerment

Mary and Dorothy both benefited from having regular contact with a centre in Tallyborough. Mary had been referred to the centre by her social worker so she could receive intensive and regular open-ended counselling:

> "She [centre worker] said to me she's not going to put any time limit. She's not going to say you an come for six weeks. She said you can come for as long as you like. She said a lot of anger will come to the surface but she said, 'I won't let you get upset'. So I'm hoping that will help." (Mary)

Often resources within the voluntary sector are much more flexible than in the statutory sector; for example, the social worker could not have given Mary as much time as the counsellor in the centre.

Dorothy found it very difficult to talk about the abuse experienced from her grandson, but knew that she could drop in to see the counsellor whenever she wanted (this tended to be around 9.00am after her grandson had left for school). It was useful for Dorothy that regular appointments were not deemed necessary as she just wanted 'someone to listen' when she was in crisis.

Trauma centres are developing around the UK to help with victims who have experienced different types of trauma (such as war, sexual abuse and so on). Such centres could be of help to victims of elder abuse.

One idea welcomed by victims was having a special trauma centre for victims of elder abuse where the following could be provided:

- Emergency beds
- Drop-in/day-care facilities – to be used when and as the victim wished
- Sessions/surgeries to be provided by:
  - counsellors – to cover a wide rage of counselling needs;
  - therapists;
  - solicitor;
  - DSS officer;
  - social worker;
  - housing officer;
  - doctor;
  - nurse.
- Education/training courses
- Library

Whatever centre is used to help the victim, proper introductions and support are important. A victim's self-esteem may be low, and walking into a new environment may be very frightening:

"I need my confidence back. I might get it back by attending the bingo session or coffee mornings on a Monday at the community centre which is just across from the bungalow.... I mean the thought of walking into that community centre terrified me at first it really did and then I started to think – well I'm getting used to the fact that I am with new people so I am going to have to get to know these people that I live amongst and the other warden she put it to me – 'Why don't you just pop over some Monday morning?'. She said, 'There is not a big crowd on a Monday morning and just get talking to a few of them'." (Vera)

Day care and community centres

Day care can be invaluable in supporting the victim in both practical and emotional ways:

- Social activities
- Personal care – for example bathing facilities, hairdresser (which can also be important in building self-esteem)
- Healthcare – physiotherapists, occupational therapists, speech therapists, dieticians
- Food and warmth
- Company

When a victim receives regular day care, staff may need to:

- Listen
- Support
- Receive disclosure
- Report
- Offer advice
- Make referrals for specialist advice/support/counselling/therapy

Community centres can also be an important source of social activity; this was particularly so for Isabella, who attended three days a week and she said she liked 'making friends' and the 'coffee mornings'. Jessie felt that a community centre would benefit the people living in her area:

"We haven't got a social centre on this estate at all and when it was first built it was in the plans that the centre would be built … a community centre, and where the shops are that's where it was, but they reckon they have no space now to do it and there is plenty of space. There is plenty of holes that they can put it in so that is a poor excuse in my eyes." (Jessie)

Hobbies and interests

Loneliness is one of the most common difficulties presented by victims. Thus, company, social activities and outings can be very important, but, again, it must be emphasised that assessment of this may take time. It should not be assumed that every older person likes playing bingo or dominoes and watching old films. The assessor must find what interests the individual victim:

> "I love to read Mills and Boon. I have a box full here." (Joan)

> "I watch television and I read. I like Maeve Binchy ... I can't handle a hardback with my arthritis in my hands.... They keep buying me video tapes ... I have asked for Titanic ... and for Cliff Richard in Wuthering Heights." (Daphne)

Outings are important in order to keep contact with the outside world. Almost all of the victims interviewed said they had enjoyed going to the local market to shop when they were younger and this was part of their routine; organised outings to shops were welcomed. This was particularly important to Georgina once she had been placed in permanent residential care – she enjoyed being taken to new large shopping centres and being pushed around the shops in her wheelchair by care staff. For victims still living in the community, outings organised by centres may be the only way of getting out socially.

Many older people are illiterate and may want to learn to read and write; they may have other unfulfilled ambitions. Creative writing enables some victims to vent their feelings about what has happened. It was noted earlier that some victims choose to disclose by writing notes to indicate that they want help to get out of the situation. For some victims, writing can be a way of healing. Vera continued to write a diary after she had left her husband.

Education and training can be important to older people and opportunities should be offered whenever possible. This could involve skills development to help them develop confidence, such as assertiveness courses, or courses which develop their interests or hobbies.

"We are doing glass painting and woodwork. There is a group just started doing manicures ... I have just taken a course on peer support." (Jessie)

Other problems

Some victims may have long-standing problems which need to be worked on. Lilian had had a drink problem for over 30 years – a common strategy for victims trying to cope with abuse. This was well documented on her files and staff in the resource centre had started to address this with Lilian. However, as soon as she was placed in a nursing home, nothing was followed up. A proper assessment of the problem should have been undertaken and discussed with Lilian herself, getting her placed seemed to take priority over resolving the long-term problem of heavy drinking.

Physical help

It is important to assess health needs and it should be remembered that these may change over time. Some disabled victims will need help with personal care, or there may be other medical problems which require attention, so there may be a role for home care, district nurses, community psychiatric nurses and so on. A victim who has experienced physical or sexual abuse may find it difficult to accept any help which involves direct contact with her body and helpers need to acknowledge this. A victim may also appear obsessional about washing and have excessively high standards of hygiene. Some victims may have conditions which cause them physical pain because of injuries incurred; skin conditions are common among victims. Consequently, if engaging in personal care tasks, helpers need to treat the victim with care and sensitivity.

Company

It was suggested that centres can help towards addressing the problem of loneliness (see above), but some individuals do not like being part of a group. For some victims it will be necessary to establish support in a one-to-one situation. Outreach work is important and can be undertaken by volunteers, befrienders or the establishment of 'buddy schemes'.

Practical help

> ### The following practical resources were advocated by victims:
>
> - Personal alarms
> - Alarm systems linked to someone
> - Closed circuit television cameras
> - Telephone
> - Entry telephones (to sheltered accommodation)
> - List of useful telephone numbers
> - Local police telephone numbers
> - Leaflets with information.

Safety

It will be apparent that most of the practical help requested by victims in interviews and focus groups were related to safety issues and maintaining contact with the outside world. It was crucial to them not only to feel safe but to be able to summon help quickly:

> "If the warden doesn't call in she calls over the intercom and it makes you feel settled." (Vera)

Some victims had personal alarms systems and found them a great comfort, but others like Bertha had refused to have this link because of the cost:

> "Yes, they came round to sell them but I never bought one … I suppose it could help but it's just an avid drain on one's resources, which are very limited." (Bertha)

Some victims did not have to pay for their alarms as they were provided via the police or Victim Support, but others, like Bertha, had to pay around £2.50 a week on top of other charges like home care. It has to be recognised that a number of older people worry a great deal about money (particularly about having enough saved to provide for their own funerals). Consequently, they might choose to go without a crucial resource because they feel they 'are not worth it'. Such important resources should be available to all victims free of charge. Similarly, many older people still do not have a telephone; it is thought to be a luxury, but could actually be a lifeline. This begs the question, if victims do not have access to a telephone how can they summon help? In any publicity, organisations must state full addresses, as some victims may need to write for help.

Security

Most victims living in sheltered accommodation complexes felt that the entry telephones were very important and made them feel in control. However, the extra need for safety in some cases is highlighted by the case of Isabella whose nephew used to wait in the bushes until he was able to slip in behind someone else entering the building. Isabella never locked her own front door, so he gained access very easily.

A recurring suggestion from participants in the focus groups was about having closed-circuit television cameras (CCTV) in their areas, as it was felt that this might ward off offenders. A common criticism of the police was that they said they could not do anything unless the offenders were caught in the act – it was suggested that CCTV would help identify the offenders, especially the gangs who regularly harassed older victims in the community. Victims who had been mugged in the street also felt that there should be more CCTVs in shopping areas and near taxi ranks and bus stops where attacks frequently occurred.

Information

Some victims wanted information about their abuser's problem(s) and information is needed about a range of different topics (such as addictions to drugs or alcohol) and services available. Joan had been proactive in getting information about things which were affecting both her husband and sister:

> "I got books about dementia. You have not got to leave or upset them.... She [sister] forgets things so I sent her all these leaflets from the hospital about dementia and Alzheimer's disease. It could be the start of something. She ought to go to the doctor's." (Joan)

Peer support groups

Older people traditionally keep things to themselves, so that the idea of attending a group to talk about the abuse they have experienced may not be welcomed initially. Involvement in other support group activities may also be rejected. Joan dismissed the idea of attending a group for relatives of drug users when her social worker suggested this. It was thought she would similarly decline to attend the focus group run for the validation of this project's findings, but in fact she readily accepted. Vera also agreed to attend after careful consideration; this was a courageous step for her as the venue was within yards of her husband's home. Both women were active participants in the group. It was particularly interesting that all the women set about the tasks of discussing the project's findings and succeeded in giving very valuable comments, but they also (with the exception of Florence) started to tell their stories again to each other – and said they found it helpful to talk to women who had similar experiences to themselves.

Florence has always found it difficult to talk about the abuse experienced from her grandson and she remained quiet during the group discussions, but it was evident to myself and the other facilitator that she was greatly affected by what Joan had to say as their abusive situations had been identical.

When organising peer support groups for older victims, some consideration must be given to the type of abuse experienced and its possible effects on other participants. Georgina, who had been a victim of financial abuse, found it very distressing to hear Joan and Vera's disclosures about physical violence and sexual abuse.

The lessons for peer support groups learnt from this group experience have been:

- Victims should be encouraged to attend peer support groups even if the idea is alien to them in the first instance.
- Victims might be more willing to attend if they can bring a support person with them (Joan wanted her social worker with her throughout the group; Vera just wanted someone to bring her to the door).
- Victims may get something positive from hearing other victims' stories.
- Consideration should be given to the types of abuse experienced and its possible effects on other participants.

Spiritual help

Religion was important to the majority of women interviewed and they wanted to maintain their contact with the church. If housebound or placed in residential care, it is crucial that arrangements are made for a vicar, priest, or other religious/spiritual person to visit when required. Some victims may choose to use this person as a counsellor rather than someone from a helping agency.

Final journeys

It is important for victims to come to terms with what has happened earlier in life and the use of reminiscence work can be useful for this. Undertaking this work is a skill which needs to be developed through specific training, otherwise the helper may find themselves dealing with disclosures which they find difficult to handle. Some victims of elder abuse wish to revisit places which have unresolved emotive issues for them, or may need to visit places that hold happy memories. When Agnes began thinking about moving to another nursing home she thought about living at the seaside. She had happy memories of Bridlington and felt, because it is flat, she might be able to get out on her motorised wheelchair:

> "You see I know Bridlington fairly well ... there is a good crossing across the road. I would feel safe doing that and I have imagined it lots of times. You are not forced to be on the move all the time. You can just sit and look at the sea and I can talk to people if there was someone sitting close by, especially if they were sitting on their own, I can start a conversation. If they show signs of not wanting to talk then fair enough, but sometimes you can sit and have a good hour's conversation with someone." (Agnes)

Because Isabella had spent 20 years in a mental institution she often felt trapped and that she had missed out on a lot of things. She had been to Ireland once but said: "I would have liked to have gone to Germany – I did ask to go". At the time of interview Isabella's social worker was trying to organise a holiday for her later in the year, but was having problems finding a carer to go with her – this has since been resolved.

Conclusion

The needs of victims must be reassessed on a regular basis as it is likely that they will change during the short- and long-term periods when work is being undertaken. Different resources may be needed as the victim moves on or as different needs arise in the future. It is important that all workers endeavour to provide resources appropriate to the individual needs of the victims.

Overall, consideration must be given to:

- Individuality
- Short- and long-term resources
- Changing needs
- Provision/publicity of information
- Choice
- Sufficient time

8
Proper endings

All of us, as we get older, need to prepare for death, that is, to come to terms with unresolved issues before we die. 'Proper endings' are also important at interim stages of life – not least to the victims who have left abusive situations. For victims of abuse, it is often necessary to 'finish things off' and 'make a clean break'. This final chapter gives an overview of the important endings for the women interviewed in this study.

For 19 of the 27 women interviewed, abuse has stopped either because the victim chose to leave the situation, took positive action to stop the abuse, or the abuser had left. However, family members are still abusing seven women who choose to stay in their situations. Eva is adamant that the abuse has stopped but admits that there is always the fear it will start again; staff at the day centre believe that she is still being abused but is in denial. Hilda is in a similar situation. Rose continues to be harassed by gangs of youths in her area and is angry that the police still do not take the problem seriously.

For some victims who have left abusive husbands, one way of ending things properly has been to finalise the break by obtaining a divorce. At the time of writing seven women have obtained a divorce or are in the process of doing so. For some, the death of the abuser was the final break, even though they were already divorced:

> "I got divorced but he died not long after so I had wasted my time and money.... Do you know, I was glad when he died ... I was really glad." (Margaret)

During interviews women spoke about wanting to put the past behind them, but were at the same time realistic about 'needing to sort things out'. This was true for them in a practical sense, but also emotionally. This emphasises one of the most important findings of the project: that women need to come to terms with what has happened to them, to work through their feelings and then to heal. The process is exactly the same as for younger victims, but in some cases, where abuse has been experienced much earlier in life as well as recently, there is much more to address. Skilled listening and support is needed to work on these issues and specialised help may be required to work on the long-term effects of abuse, both emotional and physical. A worrying finding is that, for some women, health problems resulting from previous abuse have remained untreated. It is clear that appropriate complementary services need to be engaged in joint work towards achieving positive endings, that is, that the victim can 'move on' emotionally. Services need to be planned in a coordinated way and under the care management system this should be achievable.

Another important finding is that, for most, it is never too late to change, and this message must be spread to workers in all agencies. It is discriminatory to believe that it is not worth spending money on resources which would help older people because they may die in the near future. It is an indictment on a generation of politicians and policy makers that the old are often dismissed as an economic burden on society. Older people have a moral right to access the services they need. This project has shown that a wide range of services could help victims of abuse in both the short and long term. It is unfortunate that although a number of the women interviewed were efficiently helped to *leave* an abusive situation, no future plans for longer-term work were made to address their outstanding personal and social needs. Lilian is a prime example: she has suffered horrendous abuse throughout her life from many people, most of her 17 children have died or are in prison, and she has an alcohol problem. She has been placed in a private nursing home but is unlikely to receive any support from a counsellor or therapist. Certainly there are no plans for this additional help. What chance is there of 'proper endings' for Lilian? For some victims opportunities for proper endings are currently not available. In other cases long-term work is being undertaken. Vera continues to value the weekly counselling sessions she has with her social worker; Isabella is well supported by her social worker who has been involved with her case for four years; Gwen continues to talk to her volunteer. However, it seems that relevant service provision is somewhat hit and miss.

In some cases, experts are needed to work with victims in the long term, but a very wide range of workers are likely to encounter initial disclosures of abuse, assume responsibility for monitoring situations, and give friendly and sensible support in the long term. Thus, it is essential that agencies in all sectors – statutory, voluntary and independent – should provide training for all levels of staff, so that they are confident in skilled listening and hence in facilitating disclosure, and in offering support in both the short and long term. Many workers have never received a basic awareness training on abuse, may not be aware of what to look for, or how to support a victim in the various stages of their needs.

A 'proper ending' for the project is that the majority of victims interviewed have left their abusive situations and are safe. Perhaps one of the happiest endings has been for Agnes, whose husband had continued to emotionally abuse her in the nursing homes and then in sheltered accommodation until he died very recently. On her husband's death Agnes' son came from Australia and Agnes has now decided that she wants to put everything behind her and start a new life in Australia. All the professionals involved have done everything to support her in making this decision, and she is about to go into hospital "to be built up" for the 36-hour flight.

Many victims have regrets, although this is mainly related to the fact that they wish they had acted earlier. Victims were asked what advice they would give to other older women currently living in an abusive situation. Their messages were similar:

"If I had my time to come over again I should have pulled it up straight away. I should have stopped it straight away ... because once they get away with it, then it goes from small amounts, bigger amounts and so on and so on." (Daphne)

"When I left him I thought, 'I ought to have done this years ago'." (Margaret)

"I would tell her to walk away while she could and to make a new life for herself and it is possible. The children would be better

> without the abuse because children learn from abuse ... the young child sees what is going on to be right. The older child learns what to do to gain control of someone. So I would honestly say to anyone who is the position I was in in the early years to get up and go." (Vera)

> "Develop. To cope with it. It takes a long time to recognise it. You have got to keep trying and that's the only way you can cope with it. Telling yourself that you will get out of it. Everybody is different. You move on. You just realise one day that you don't need it. You can be you." (Mary)

> "Well, try not to show them that you are afraid, because the more you are the more they take advantage of you. Try to make out it's not affecting you." (Eva)

> "Try not to hold it in. Tell somebody. However hard it is tell somebody even if it is your best friend. Tell somebody." (Jessie)

The victims talked about the happiness they were now experiencing – happiness to which perhaps they did not think they were entitled earlier in life, but later felt they had a right to:

> "I have never been as happy as I am now, away from it." (Margaret)

> "I liked it at [residential home] ... I loved it there. I suppose it was the first time I had experienced any happiness." (Beatrice)

> "I am fine. I have been fine since I have been in here [sheltered accommodation].... Everyone here – the wardens and assistant wardens – are kindness itself." (Joan)

At a time when services are judged by outputs of change in the social functioning of service users, it seems odd to assert that happiness may also be something to strive for. As far as older victims of abuse are concerned, happiness is a legitimate goal. Certainly, some of the respondents, with the help of various workers, have found happiness, and have shown that it is never too late to 'move on' and to make 'proper endings' to earlier events in stressful lives. The challenges they pose to services are how to improve the protection of victims, how to respond at the right pace and with the right skills, and how to look to realistic futures.

References

ADSS (Association of Directors of Social Services) (1991) *Adults at risk*, Stockport: ADSS.

Aitken, L. and Griffin, G. (1996) *Gender issues in elder abuse*, London: Sage Publications.

Dixon, A. (1982) *A woman in your own right*, London: Quartet Books.

Dobash, R.E. and Dobash, R.P. (1992) *Women, violence and social change*, London: Routledge.

DoH (Department of Health)/SSI (Social Services Inspectorate) (1992) *Confronting elder abuse*, London: HMSO.

DoH/SSI (Social Services Inspectorate) (1993) *No longer afraid*, London: HMSO.

Eastman, M. (1984) *Old age abuse*, London: Age Concern.

Gelles, R.J. and Cornell, C.P. (1985) *Intimate violence in families*, Beverley Hills, CA: Sage Publications.

Hunt, L., Marshall, M. and Rowlings, C. (1997) *Past trauma in later life*, London: Jessica Kingsley Publishers.

McCreadie, M. (1996) *Elder abuse: Update on research*, London: Institute of Gerontology, Kings College.

Maykut, P. and Morehouse, R. (1994) *Beginning qualitative research: A philosophic and practical guide*, London: Falmer Press.

Morgan, D.L. (1997) *Focus groups as qualitative research* (2nd edn), Thousand Oaks, CA: Sage Publications.

Pritchard, J. (1989) 'Confronting the taboo of the abuse of elderly people', *Social Work Today*, 5 October, pp 12-13.

Pritchard, J. (1990) 'Old and abused', *Social Work Today*, 15 February, pp 22-3.

Pritchard, J. (1993) 'Gang warfare', *Community Care Magazine*, 8 July, pp 22-3.

Pritchard, J. (1995). *The abuse of older people* (2nd edn), London: Jessica Kingsley Publishers.

Pritchard, J. (1997) *The Vulnerable Adults Project: Report on initial findings*, Unpublished paper.

Pritchard, J. (1999) *Elder abuse work: Best practice in Britain and Canada*, London: Jessica Kingsley Publishers.

Appendix A: Categories of abuse

Below is a summary of the categories of abuse as defined in policies and working documents in Churchtown, Millfield and Tallyborough, which workers were asked to use when completing monitoring forms.

Physical abuse
- Bodily assaults resulting in injuries: bruises; cuts; lacerations; fractures; dislocations; wounds; physical restraint; slap marks; kick marks; black eyes; bitemarks; burns.
- Infliction of physical pain or injury; force feeding; shaking or slapping; involuntary isolation and physical confinement; administration of inappropriate drugs.
- Deliberate bodily impairment, for example, malnutrition, dehydration.
- Medical/healthcare maltreatment, for example, inappropriate medication; deliberate over/under medication

Emotional abuse
- Persistent undermining of self-esteem: humiliation; ridicule; harassment; bullying; intimidation; threats; harsh and reiterated criticism; being criticised; causing fear/mental anguish.
- Verbal attacks, for example, shouting, swearing.
- Unreasonable demands; deliberate ignoring; emotional blackmail.
- Deprivation of social contact, for example, through acts of omission or commission on the part of others, including involuntary withdrawal of a person from a valued activity.
- Persistent violation of rights normally accorded to individuals as citizens, such as choice, opinion, privacy.

Financial abuse
- Material exploitation, for example, misuse of a person's money, property, possessions, pension book or insurance, or blocking access to these material goods.
- Theft or fraud.
- Personal exploitation by misappropriation of money or goods.
- Unauthorised extraction of money or goods, for example, withdrawing money from an account; attempting to gain property against the will of a vulnerable adult; refusal to pay bills.

Neglect

- Physical neglect of the person to such an extent that health, development, well-being is impaired. This may include malnutrition, dehrydration, rashes, pressure sores.
- The withholding of adequate care for daily living to the individual: being left in wet or soiled clothing/inappropriate clothing; lack of food/drink/warmth; lack of attention to personal hygiene needs; untreated medical problems
- Deliberate refusal to meet basic needs; deprivation of nutrition; failure to assist in performing daily living tasks.
- Isolation; lack of stimulation; restricted movement; absence of mobility aids.
- Environmental abuse, such as, no light, no ventilation, inadequate space.

Sexual abuse

- The involvement of adults in sexual activities without their informed consent or where the individual has insufficient mental capacity to have full understanding of the activity.
- Inappropriate touching; fondling; kissing; oral contact; genital contact; digital penetration (vagina or anus); rape; penetration with objects; exploitation; forced exposure to or involvement in pornography; ritual/satanic abuse.

Appendix B: The interviewees

Victim	Age	Type of elder abuse	Abuser(s)	Previous abuse	Substantial references
Agnes	78	PEF	Husband	CA/DV	40, 44-5, 48-9, 52, 61, 69, 97, 107, 111
Beatrice	91	F	Carer/gangs (M)	CA(M)	41, 66, 68, 70-1, 112
Bertha	91	F	Carer	?CA	41, 67, 104
Catherine	60	PEF	Son-in-law		62, 68, 90
Daphne	79	F	Granddaughter		43, 63, 65, 70, 102, 111
Dorothy	62	PE	Grandson		99-100
Emma	80	PEF	Husband	DV	40, 44, 48, 53, 55-60, 89, 94
Ethel	95	PEN (?S)	Son		46
Eva	77	PEF	Husband/son (M)	DV	44, 51, 109, 112
Florence	80	PEF	Grandson		41, 106
Georgina	85	F	Stranger		69-70, 102, 106
Gertrude	92	F	Neighbour		72
Gwen	98	F	Step-daughter	CA/DV	68-9, 110
Harriet	90	S	Neighbour	CA/?DV	46-7, 63
Hilda	64	EF	Son	DV	49-50, 66, 71, 109
Irene	84	PF	Two sons/grandson		41-2, 55
Isabella	76	EF	Carer/nephew (M)	DV	41, 45, 67, 107, 110
Jessie	54	EFS	Stranger/brother (M)	CA/DV	47, 51-2, 73, 91-2, 98, 101, 103, 112
Joan	78	PEF	Grandson		41-2, 49, 51, 57, 89, 93, 102, 105-6, 112
Lilian	73	PEF	Son	CA/DV	49, 56-7, 71, 103, 110

Victim	Age	Type of elder abuse	Abuser(s)	Previous abuse	Substantial references
Margaret	81	PE	Husband	DV	40, 48, 54, 65, 98, 109, 111-12
Martha	81	F	Son/daughter/ stranger	DV	43-4, 48, 51, 72-3, 92
Mary	60	PE	Husband	CA/DV	97-9, 112
Rose	81	EF	Gangs		73, 92, 109
Sarah	81	PEN	Sister		46, 51
Stella	89	E	Husband/family		46, 62, 67
Vera	63	PEFNS	Husband	DV	45, 47-50, 56, 59-60, 64, 71, 89, 91, 94-5, 97, 100-101, 104, 106, 110-12

Key: P = physical; E = emotional; F = financial; N = neglect; S = sexual; ?=suspected abuse; M = multiple victim; CA = child abuse; DV = domestic violence.